METRONOMIC PHYTONUTRITION

How daily, regular intake of plant-based foods may decrease cancer risk

Mark A. Marinella, MD, FACP

Board certified: Internal Medicine and Medical Oncology
Dayton Physicians Network
Assistant Clinical Professor of Internal Medicine
Wright State University School of Medicine
Dayton, Ohio

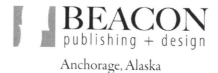

BEACON
publishing + design

Anchorage, Alaska

More Praise for "Metronomic Phytonutrition"

"Everyone reading Dr. Marinella's book will benefit from his wisdom. A must read for practical advice to easily incorporate great-tasting phytonutrient-rich foods daily. *Metronomic Phytonutrition* is research-based and well documented."
– *Debra Thompson MS, RDN, LD, Oncology Dietitian, Dayton, OH*

"Studies continue to show direct correlations between nutrition, general health and disease survival. Nowhere is this more important than in the development of holistic treatment processes for cancer care. Kudos to Dr. Marinella for providing this timely and tremendously valuable resource. It is sure to become a mainstay in our fight against this terrible disease."
– *Mark W. Moronell, MD FACC, VP of Cardiovascular Service Line Premier Health, Dayton, OH*
Author of "An Overview of the Medical Landscape"

"The National Cancer Institute in 2016 validated that good nutrition is important for cancer patients, that healthy eating habits are important during cancer treatment, that cancer can change the way the body uses food, thus drawing the potential line between cancer, its treatment, and the importance of healthy nutrition to improve outcomes. As an advanced practice nurse for the last 25 years, I have personally observed the impact of nutrition on cancer patients. It has also been my observation working alongside Dr. Mark Marinella, that he is a tireless, innovative, research-focused medical oncologist and his research and application of discovered best practice in this area of nutrition are without rival. Thus, I would quickly endorse anything penned by Dr. Marinella regarding the correlation between cancer, cancer treatment and the impact of nutrition."

– *Elizabeth Delaney, DNP, CNS, OCN, ACHNP, Nurse Practitioner at Dayton Physicians Network, Assistant Professor of Nursing, School of Nursing, Cedarville University*

"Diet plays an important role in the causation or decreasing the risk of cancer. Dr. Mark Marinella, a renowned medical oncologist, did extensive literature review for writing this book to make it as much evidence-based as possible. I found it very informative and insightful."
– *Satheesh Kathula, MD, FACP, Clinical Professor of Medicine Wright State University School of Medicine*
Board of Trustees, American Association of Physicians from Indian Origin
Advisor, Multicultural Center for Excellence, Pfizer

"A top notch recipe for well-being and health, where exercise and nutrition are key ingredients for disease management and prevention! Dr. Marinella cleverly combines the art and science of food nutrition in this highly informative book for clinicians and patients alike. Bon appetit!"
– *Christine Broomhall, MS, BSN, RN, ACSM-CES, Miami Valley Hospital, Dayton, OH*
Cardiovascular and Pulmonary Rehabilitation, Premier HeartWorks

"Dr. Marinella has been my physician since the discovery of my stage four lymphoma four years ago. Under his care, I went into remission within a year and am still in remission. When I say 'under his care' this includes not only chemotherapy, but also his advice to lead a full life and assure proper nutrition. My wife, also a cancer survivor, and I have each read his enjoyable and thoroughly researched book, *Metronomic Phytonutrition*, in detail. It is readily understood by the lay person and has led us to significantly change our approach to our diet. We have learned about phytonutrients and the surprising medical benefits of the right blend of foods while avoiding the need for expensive supplements which can sometimes be unsafe when faced with the necessity to take prescription drugs. Through Dr. Marinella's guidance and his encouragement to educate ourselves in phytonutrition, my wife and I are enjoying foods that are delicious as well as healthy. Anyone who has to take on the adventure of surviving cancer deserves the opportunity that Dr. Marinella's book provides to win deliciously while perhaps adding more exciting years to their lives. Furthermore, I strongly recommend this book to even those who do not have cancer. What he describes and recommends is a nutritional lifestyle designed to help avoid cancer as much as aid in the recovery. I have never enjoyed food more and I know that what I am eating is helping me to win!"
– *Tom Ireland, Dayton, OH*

*"Let food be thy medicine
and medicine be thy food."*

Hippocrates

`

METRONOMIC PHYTONUTRITION:

How daily, regular intake of plant-based foods may decrease cancer risk

Copyright © 2017 by Mark Marinella, MD

Published by Beacon Publishing & Design, LLC dba Beacon Media + Marketing

3201 C Street, Ste. 302, Anchorage, Alaska 99507, 907-563-6008, printing@beaconmm.com www.beaconmm.com

Printed in the United States of America.

Cataloging-in-Publication data for this book is available from the Library of Congress.

ISBN 13: 978-0-9831644-3-2

For information and inquiries, contact Dr. Mark Marinella at mmarinella@daytonphysicians.com

Dedication

To Lana. You have given me grace, love,
steadfastness, support, and a smile since day one.
You are a gem, and I love you.

Foreword

Lifestyle interventions are widely argued by the scientific community for health promotion, prevention and treatment of non-communicable diseases (NCDs). Nutrition, as science, is one of the main pillars of Lifestyle Medicine and nowadays, thanks to progress in research, we have the opportunity to use it with greater awareness compared with the past. We have learned to appreciate foods not only for their tastes, but also for their content of functional substances.

Since the 1980s, the focus of Western research was on identifying and understanding those chemicals, termed nutrients, that are needful for health and survival. There has been a large discussion about the essentialness of nutrients, and this discussion is reflected in the changing approach to the establishment of human nutrient reference standards. In the Far East, emphasis has been focused on using the nonnutrient chemicals in plant parts for medicinal treatment. In the past 20 years, these 2 concepts have begun to merge, as Western countries examine nonnutritive plant constituents as sources of health benefits.

Also known as phytochemicals, these bioactive constituents aren't real essential nutrients (that is essential for development, growth and maintenance of our body), and provide even less energy (they have no "calories"). We are talking, however, about substances capable of modulating several biological activities and important functions of the body, such as the antioxidant and anti-inflammatory activity, modulation of detoxification enzymes, stimulation of the immune system, modulation of the hormonal metabolism and antibacterial and antiviral activity, etc.

i

The concept of *Metronomic Phytonutrition*, here presented by Mark A. Marinella M.D., admirably expresses the need of human physiology to be constantly supported and sustained by phytochemicals to ensure adequate survival of our species in this inhuman world.

There is still much to clarify about the biological activity, the bioavailability in food and the metabolism of phytochemicals. To paraphrase Dr. Marinella, is that a mostly plant diet may decrease the incidence of NCDs in a safe manner while providing other benefits such as improving subjective well-being and enjoying the wonderful taste of this type of dietary pattern.

Luigi Maselli, MD
Scientific Director - National Department of Lifestyle Sciences – Italy
Member of International Board of Lifestyle Medicine

Acknowledgements

I wish to thank those who reviewed my manuscript and kindly offered endorsements—I know how valuable your time is and I greatly appreciate your willingness. I also wish to extend gratitude to Adrienne, Jennifer, and the design team at Beacon Publishing & Design for their insight and foresight for this book as well as their wonderful skills at publishing, layout, and cover design.

Table of Contents

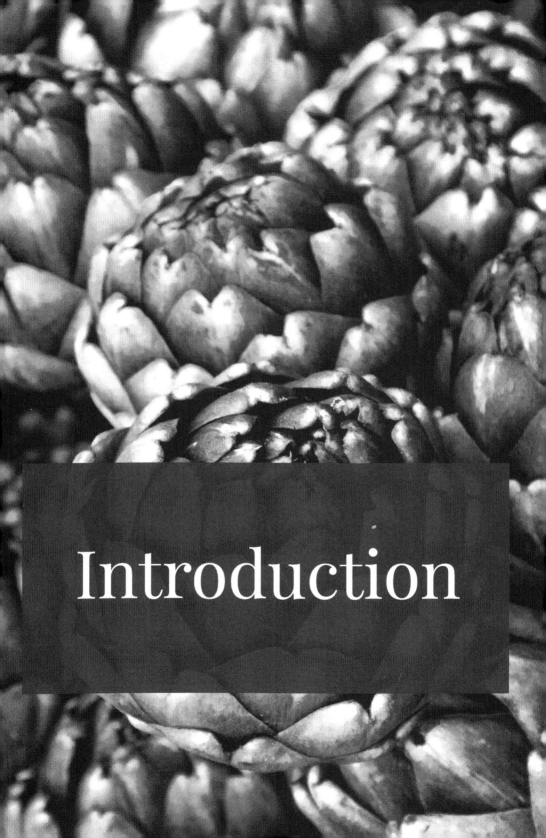

Introduction

As a practicing medical oncologist, I see dozens of patients with cancer during a typical work week. No one can know for certain what role, if any, nutrition or diet has played in the causation of any person's individual cancer. Since cancer is a very complicated process that involves genetics, environmental exposures, and spontaneous, unpredictable cell and/or DNA damage, pinning the etiology of a specific cancer on a poor diet is very difficult. That being stated, however, it is clear from numerous published studies, that diet contributes to a significant percentage of a variety of cancers worldwide. Indeed, some cancers such as colorectal cancer are very uncommon in many African countries and India—a phenomenon most likely related to high dietary intake of fiber in the form of vegetables, fruits, and grains as well as the antioxidant content of certain spices, herbs, and seeds in these populations. The medical literature is becoming replete with articles and studies on the protective role that plant-based foods play in decreasing the risk of chronic illness.[1] Indeed, plant-based diets and remedies have been utilized for millennia to prevent and treat various ailments and various plants have been developed into not only complimentary treatments but also therapeutic drugs such as antimicrobials and chemotherapy.[2]

This book, *Metronomic Phytonutrition: How daily, regular intake of plant-based foods may decrease cancer risk*, was borne out of my passion for taking care of cancer patients and my personal interest in Mediterranean-style cooking. The use of a variety of vegetables, fruits, seeds, nuts, herbs, and spices in daily meal preparation provides significant amounts of "phytonutrients" — plant-derived chemicals that can have dramatic health-promoting properties, including cancer prevention (the term phytonutrient and phytochemical are

---

1 Ferrari CK, Perario S, Silva JC, et al. *An apple plus a Brazil nut a day keeps the doctors away: antioxidant capacity of foods and their health benefits.* Curr Pharm Des 2016;22:189-195
2 Fridlender M, Kapulnik Y, Koltai H. *Plant-derived substances with anticancer activity: from folklore to practice.* Front Plant Sci 2016;6:799-808

synonymous and are used interchangeably in this book). By combining my interests in medical oncology and cooking, I devised the concept *"metronomic phytonutrition"* which, as will be explained in detail later in this book, is the long-term, regular consumption of phytonutrient-enriched foods. I posit that this may favorably impact health by not only possibly lowering an individual's risk of certain cancers, but also by decreasing the incidence of some malignancies on a population-wide level. Of course, diet does *not* guarantee that one will not get cancer. However, it may decrease risk in a safe manner while providing other benefits such as improving subjective well-being, decreasing the incidence of cardiovascular disease, and enjoying the wonderful taste of this type of dietary pattern.

My end-goal of this book is to present the concept of *"metronomic phytonutrition"* to everyone, hoping that these principles will be "added on" to whatever diet they currently pursue, in hopes of sparking interest in nutrition and its role in disease prevention.

Mark A. Marinella, MD, FACP
Dayton, OH
May 2017

Note From the Author

Although I am a firm believer in good nutrition and the role that it plays in preventing disease and maintaining health, I am also a strong proponent of modern medical therapy. Medicine has evolved significantly over the last few decades thanks to not only practicing physicians, but also to academic physicians, researchers, the pharmaceutical industry, and other scientists. Indeed, in the field of cancer medicine, we have recently witnessed an explosion of therapies for historically difficult-to-treat cancers such as melanoma, lung cancer, and kidney cancer. We as oncologists are now starting to routinely administer agents known as "checkpoint inhibitors" that stimulate the body's own immune cells to attack cancer and, although not all patients experience a favorable response, many patients have experienced amazing benefits unheard of only a few years ago. Additionally, numerous advancements in chemotherapy, oral anticancer drugs, surgery, radiation, and supportive care have improved outcomes for many cancer patients with more tolerable side effects.

That all being stated, there is ample data that some cancers may be preventable with a diet rich in plant-based foods that is low in red and processed meats. Also, a "favorable lifestyle" pattern that includes adequate intake of a plant-based diet and regular exercise, decreases risk of cardiovascular disease, as shown recently in a study published in the *New England Journal of Medicine*.[1] Good nutrition during treatment of cancer and other diseases also may enhance well-being and make some therapies more tolerable. However, in regards to treatment of cancer and many other chronic disease states, nutrition alone does not constitute, nor is it a substitute for, adequate modern medical treatment.

---

1 *Khera AV, Emdin CA, Drake I, et al. Genetic risk, adherence to a healthy lifestyle, and coronary disease. N Engl J Med 2016;375:2349-2358*

No part of this book is meant to diagnose or treat cancer or any disease or to substitute for the advice of a physician. I also suggest checking with one's physician before embarking on any major dietary changes in order to avoid any interactions with diet and medications (e.g., the effect of the blood thinner warfarin may be blunted by ingestion of certain leafy greens rich in vitamin K).

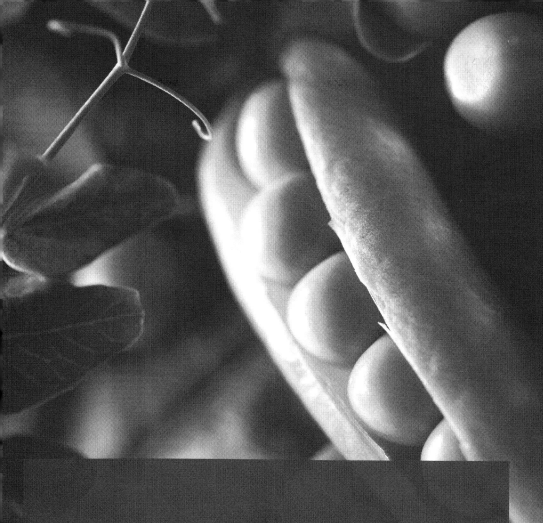

Chapter I
Another Nutrition Book?

Why another book on food and nutrition? Indeed, strolling through the local bookstore, one finds a plethora of books on dieting or the latest fad on how to improve health, stop disease in its tracks, and guarantee weight loss — all while having abundant energy! While many exaggerated claims are made in books, magazines, websites, and social media outlets, our culture is realizing the importance of a healthy diet as it relates to well-being. However, chronic illness such as cardiovascular disease and cancer claim numerous lives annually — some of which are probably preventable. While inherent genetic makeup of an individual determines health to an undeniable degree, diet does play an important role in the prevention of disease.

First, certain nutrients are vital to prevent the development of certain deficiency states or diseases such as marasmus (protein deficiency), scurvy (vitamin C deficiency), and rickets (vitamin D deficiency). These diseases are uncommon in the Western World where food is present in abundance, and supplies adequate calories, protein, vitamins, and minerals to ward off many deficiency-related illnesses. People who develop scurvy can be treated with vitamin C with reversal of symptoms and those with marasmus can be nourished back to health by very careful administration of protein and a balanced diet. These are examples of how deficiency diseases are treated by supplying the deficient nutrient, usually a vitamin or mineral. However, in a relatively healthy and well-fed population (such as those living in Westernized countries), supplementation with extra or "supranormal" amounts of protein or vitamins does not necessarily prevent disease, and may indeed be harmful as recent studies have shown.[1-3] For instance, a clinical trial of vitamin A supplementation actually *increased* the risk of certain cancers and vitamin E supplements *increased* the risk of prostate cancer.[2] In fact, very little, if any, solid data exists that taking supplements in addition to usual diet, decreases the risk of developing cancer. [1,3]

As a practicing medical oncologist, seeing patients with early and advanced-staged cancers is a way-of-life. Some of these cancers are lifestyle-related and preventable, such as many (but NOT all) cases of lung cancer. Many cancers, however, develop in people who have "done everything right" so to speak, when it comes to avoiding smoking, exercising, and eating healthy. Cancer is a very complex process and not one disease with one cause and one cure. Indeed, there is no solitary "magic bullet" cure for cancer in general, or for any one cancer type, specifically. For instance, breast cancer is a very common cancer but a very heterogeneous disease with multiple subtypes that are treated differently and have different prognoses.

For some cancers, there are well-described "targets" that can be honed in on with various available drugs—this is known to oncologists as "targeted therapy." For example, about 20% of breast cancers harbor an abnormal amount of a gene called HER2-*neu*. Tumors that express this "target" can have dramatic responses to a drug known as traztuzumab (Herceptin®), a drug that has improved prognosis significantly for women with this subtype of breast cancer. Similarly, an uncommon cancer known as chronic myeloid leukemia (CML) almost always carries an abnormal gene rearrangement known as BCR-ABL. This "target" is treated with one of a few oral drugs on the market: imatinib (Gleevec®), dasatinib (Sprycel®), or nilotinib (Tasigna®); all of these drugs result in dramatic improvement for the patient, often to the point that it is nearly impossible to detect a trace of disease! However, patients with HER2 positive breast cancer and BCR-ABL positive CML can develop resistance to these medicines, allowing the cancer to start growing and spreading again. This is because the tumor cells develop complex growth pathways to outsmart the drug. If one considers all of the different types of cancer (well over 100) and that each individual cancer consists of billions of cells that can mutate, it is easy to understand why there is no single cure for cancer. As such, prevention of cancer to any degree within a population can have a large impact on that nation's health. What if 10% of cases of a certain type of cancer could be prevented with diet? If there were 100,000 annual new cases of that particular cancer, then 10,000 people would not develop that cancer! So, we need to pay attention to diet and its ability to prevent some cancers, while realizing not all cancers will be prevented.

Treating established cancer requires multiple modalities that may include surgery, radiation, chemotherapy, and newer biologic and immune-stimulating drugs. The ingestion of dietary supplements during active anticancer therapy may indeed be harmful, especially if high doses of antioxidants such as vitamins C or E are taken, as these may impair the effects of chemotherapy or radiation. Herbal supplements may affect drug metabolism thereby increasing the risk of drug toxicity or potentially negating the effects of anticancer drugs. Many drugs and herbs are metabolized in the liver through a system known as *cytochrome P-450*, which may activate or detoxify the particular agent. As such, given the complexity of modern cancer drugs, many oncologists have concerns about patients taking herbs or other dietary supplements during cancer treatment. Indeed, researchers recently published in the journal *Blood*, that high amounts of green tea ingestion actually interfere with the action of a widely used cancer drug known as bortezomib (Velcade®), used to treat a blood cancer known as multiple myeloma. [4] This certainly speaks against using capsules containing green tea extract during treatment with this drug.

This book is NOT meant to address nutrition or supplementation for patients under active cancer treatment. This book is also NOT a diet book or a "magic" formula for guaranteeing a life free of cancer. Rather, it presents a pragmatic idea that relates to our daily diet and how adopting a lifestyle of relatively simple food additions may decrease

cancer risk. I have tried to base as much as possible on published medical literature. I will

be the first to attest, however, that much of the data regarding cancer and diet is based

on *in vitro* laboratory and animal experiments. However, several epidemiologic and

population-based studies clearly show an inverse association between ingestion of certain

plants and their by-products and development of certain cancers. Indeed, many cancer

drugs are plant-derived and the concept of a plant-based diet in disease prevention is not a

new idea. The Mediterranean diet is arguably the most well-known lifestyle that has been

demonstrated to decrease risk of chronic illness such as cardiovascular disease, diabetes, and

certain cancers.

 Metronomic Phytonutrition: How daily, regular intake of plant-based foods may decrease cancer risk is not meant to mimic or add to existing published books on the Mediterranean

diet. Instead, this book represents a simple concept (of a medical oncologist that loves

to cook!) based on literature, where available, that the *daily* and *consistent* intake of plant-

based foods may decrease the chances of developing certain cancers. If one is consuming

a vegetarian or Mediterranean diet, adding some or all of the foods listed in *Appendix 1* of

this book would be worthwhile—thereby increasing one's daily intake of phytonutrients.

It is well-established that certain cultures such as India have a very low risk of colorectal

cancer—a phenomena most plausibly related to not only the absence of red meat intake,

but also to the abundant daily intake of phytonutrients from protean sources such as

vegetables, fruits, seeds, and spices. Similarly, Japan boasts the longest life-span in the world

and this also likely relates to certain chronic dietary patterns. Some feel that this may be

in-part explained by mustard seed/oil intake which is very high in Japan and possesses

anticancer properties.

Metronomic Phytonutrition is a term I devised that is a hybrid of words and prefixes encountered in my livelihood as a practicing board-certified medical oncologist, my amateur endeavors as an acoustic guitar player, and a wanna-be chef. *Metronomic* refers to continuous or ongoing—the way a metronome consistently and continuously paces the beat for a musician. The term *metronomic* is almost exclusively used in the field of medical oncology, as it pertains to the administration of daily, ongoing, low-dose oral chemotherapy to treat some refractory cancers. Although not widely used, metronomic chemotherapy may have significant antitumor effects and benefit some patients. My adoption of the term *metronomic* for purposes of this book, refers to consistent, long-term (over years or a lifetime) ingestion of phytonutrient-rich foods. The root word *phyto-* basically means plant or something related to plants. Nutrition (although a word with numerous applications and contextual definitions) refers to one's basic intake of foods that make up their daily diet. Together, *phyto-* and nutrition meld a concept of plant products occupying a solid niche in the daily diet. So, to sum it up, one may now define *metronomic phytonutrition* as the consistent and ongoing ingestion of plant-derived foods, preferably with every meal.

Data is accumulating that thousands of phytochemicals present in numerous foods may decrease the risk of cellular inflammation and acquisition of a cancer phenotype by a healthy cell.[5-7] Studies have also shown that some phytochemicals can slow or stop the growth of established cancer cells *in vitro* and in animal models.[5] The ways in which the thousands of phytochemicals exert their effects is beyond the scope of this book. However, I wish to introduce the reader as to why I believe daily ingestion of phytochemical-rich foods may provide health benefits, including a lower risk of cancer. An important point to be made is that taking an individual compound as a dietary supplement does *not* provide the same benefit as obtaining that same compound in the context of the whole food. The entire "mileau" of the whole food and/or foods ingested is necessary for proper absorption, activation, and prevention of degradation of various phytonutrients.[5]   Instead, it seems from accumulating data, that taking an individual supplement is not beneficial when it comes to cancer prevention. As Liu[6] has stated, "...the additive and synergistic effects of phytochemicals in fruits and vegetables are responsible for these potent antioxidant anticancer activities and that the benefit of a diet rich in fruits and vegetables is attributed to the complex mixture of phytochemicals present in whole foods." He goes on to say that, "this explains why no single antioxidant can replace the combination of natural phytochemicals in fruits and vegetables to achieve health benefits." As such, my recommendation to patients and friends is to obtain phytonutrients from a variety of foods and spices with every meal and snack and to avoid relying on supplements. Supplements can be potentially dangerous especially if one is taking other prescription drugs. As a general rule, ingestion of plant foods is safe if done in moderation and not to excess. Phytochemicals are best obtained from a variety of sources such as vegetables, fruits, seeds, nuts, herbs and spices.

I hope this short book (meant to be read in one or two sittings to keep the reader's attention!) will foster interest into the fascinating topic of phytonutrients and the potential they hold to enhance the health of the individual as well as large populations. Most of us are blessed to have access to the foods presented in *Appendix 1* and adding them to the diet is actually quite simple—especially for the powerful spices and herbs. I favor adopting a lifestyle of consistent intake of healthy nutrient-dense foods and not necessarily a "diet." Indeed, adoption of the Mediterranean diet was found to be as effective as other commonly used "diets" for moderate weight loss. What is vital, however, is being consistent with a balanced phytonutrient-dense diet coupled with regular physical activity. The reader is referred to other books for recommendations of total caloric, fat, protein, and carbohydrate intake appropriate for their age, gender, and size.

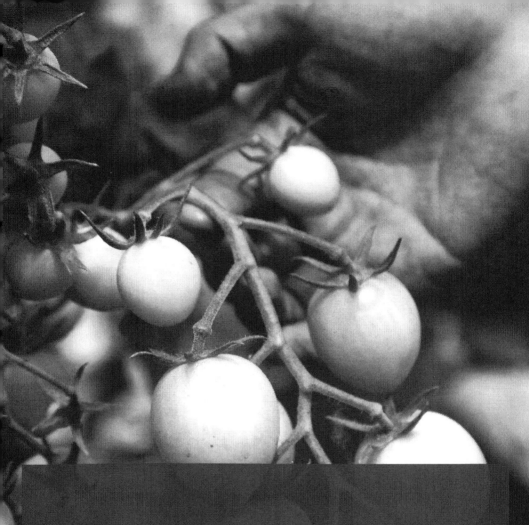

Chapter II

Nutrition and Cancer: A Brief Overview

It is well-established that cancer is a complex process with multiple contributing factors such as genetic background, habits such as smoking, environmental toxins, viruses, and diet. One cannot change their genetic predisposition to cancer, especially in cases of familial inheritance of a cancer gene (e.g., the Breast Cancer gene or BRCA). For example, women who inherit the BRCA gene have a very high risk of developing breast and/or ovarian cancer during their lifetime. This genetic change cannot be altered by any intervention, although preventative mastectomy and ovary removal significantly decreases the likelihood of contracting cancer of the breast and ovaries, respectively. However, one can avoid certain cancer-causing activities such as smoking, which is responsible for a large proportion of cancer deaths annually. Smoking is clearly associated with lung cancer as well as cancers of the oral cavity, throat, esophagus, stomach, pancreas, kidney, and bladder.

Excessive alcohol intake increases the risk of cancers of the oral cavity, esophagus, breast, and liver. Increased food intake resulting in obesity increases risk of uterine and prostate cancer—both hormone-related cancers. Environmental agents that contribute to cancer include asbestos (mesothelioma), radon (lung cancer), dyes (bladder cancer), and pesticides (lymphoma/myeloma), to name but a few. Virally-induced cancers include those due to human papillomaviruses (tonsil, cervix, and anal cancer) and hepatitis B and C (liver cancer). Some of these aforementioned risks can be avoided, others cannot. However, diet is a modifiable factor that is being increasingly shown to decrease the risk of developing some types of cancer.

From the outset, it must be stressed that a *consistent* (not perfect) and *prolonged* intake of phytonutrient-rich foods is key to lowering risk of cancer and other chronic diseases. It is well-established that many cases of cardiovascular disease are diet-related and that adoption of a "heart healthy" dietary lifestyle has significant benefits. One bad meal in the context of a *consistent* healthy diet does not ruin one's health just as one good meal in the context of a *consistent* unhealthy diet does not improve one's health. As such, diet fads and the latest supplements to induce weight loss and health are unlikely to reap significant benefits. As stated in the introduction, multivitamin and other supplements do not necessarily prevent cancer. One reason for this, is that vitamins and minerals are mainly used in the body as cofactors for various metabolic processes and supranormal intake is not necessarily better that the recommended daily allowance (RDA). Furthermore, it is the combination of various non-vitamin nutrients ingested as whole foods that seems to lower cancer risk. One compound may be important for absorption and/or activation of another nutrient and this is unlikely to be achieved with supplements.

Adoption of a plant-based diet is an important step in the prevention of cancer. Although not every cancer can be prevented even with an optimal diet, populations such as the Seventh Day Adventists, who are primarily vegetarian, have a lower risk of various cancers.[1,2] Globally, persons residing in certain parts of the Mediterranean who consume large amounts of plant-based nutrients frequently enjoy longevity.[3,4] This will be discussed in a later chapter, but it is clear that diet plays a vital role for health-enhancement on a population-wide level. Unfortunately, the typical American, "Westernized" diet often includes low amounts of fruits, vegetables, whole grains, and healthy oils. In fact, most Americans do not ingest the suggested amounts of dietary fiber and servings of fresh fruits and vegetables that have been shown to improve health. Many of our foods are processed with refined flour and sugars—which increase the risk of obesity, diabetes, cardiovascular disease, and cancer. Unhealthy oils and trans-fats found in fast- and snack foods can induce systemic inflammation which can lead to vascular and cell damage, increasing the risk of cardiovascular disease and cancer.

A diet rich in fruits and vegetables has been shown in some studies to decrease the risk of oral cavity and digestive tract cancers by up to 50%. [5-8] The combination of nutrients, rather than one individual compound or vitamin, is a common theme in population-based studies that demonstrate decreased cancer risk with fruit and vegetable intake. An excess of red meat ingestion is associated with increased risk of colorectal cancer, so limiting intake in association with adequate intake of plant-based foods, seems to be the most prudent, and simple, way of decreasing cancer risk. Additionally, certain beverages such as tea have been linked to an overall reduction in cancer risk. Green tea (see *Appendix 1*) contains several powerful antioxidants and phytochemicals that have been demonstrated to inhibit cancer cell growth and spread. Altogether, adoption of a plant-based diet seems to lower cancer risk.

A large population-based study published in the *New England Journal of Medicine* assessed over 20,000 adults living in Greece, on adherence to a Mediterranean diet and total mortality as well as cancer-related mortality.[9] Over a 44 month period, consistent adherence to a Mediterranean diet was associated with a 24% decreased risk of dying from cancer. Similar data has been published over the years that links a diet high in plant-based foods and healthy oils to a lower risk of developing cancer in general. Interestingly, people who move from countries with lower cancer risk often acquire a higher risk of cancer when moving to the United States and adopting a typical Western diet. In summary, diet seems to play an important role in the development of many cancers. Adoption of a diet similar to those residing in the Mediterranean seems to lower cancer risk based on published data.

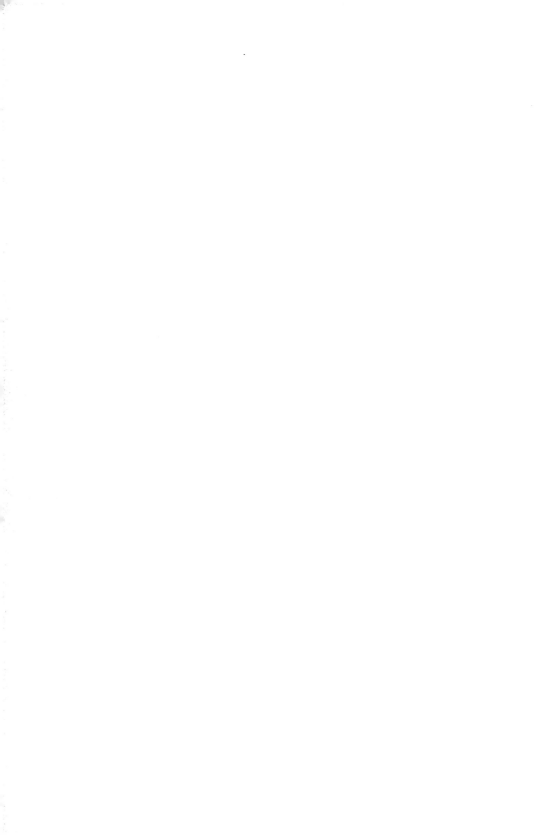

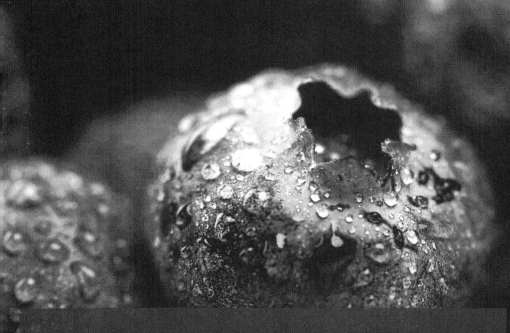

Chapter III
What Are Phytonutrients?

The word "phytonutrient" may be a new word for many people, but is an important word to understand as it relates to one's health and well-being. It is safe to assume that most people have heard the word "vitamin" since we walk past vitamin supplements in the grocery store or pharmacy and can read the recommended daily allowance (RDA) of certain vitamins on virtually every food container. While vitamins are essential, it is important to understand their role in human health and disease as well as their limitations.

Vitamins are inorganic molecules that typically act as cofactors for numerous chemical reactions that take place within cells. For instance, vitamin C (ascorbic acid) is a water-soluble vitamin that is required for proper formation of the connective tissue substance known as collagen. Collagen is vital to provide strength to blood vessels, skin, and the skeleton. Deficiency of vitamin C leads to defective and weak collagen formation that leads to bleeding, bruising, and skeletal injuries. The overt deficiency state from vitamin C deficiency is known as scurvy and is uncommon in the Western world where vitamin C-rich fruits are widely available. Although vitamin C has antioxidant properties, high doses have not been definitively shown to prevent cancer and may lead to adverse effects such as stomach irritation and kidney stones. Similarly, thiamine (vitamin B1) is a water-soluble vitamin that is an important cofactor for a variety of metabolic reactions that metabolize sugars and carbohydrates. Deficiency of thiamine leads to the disease *beri-beri*, which is characterized by heart failure, swelling, nerve damage and, if untreated, death. *Beri-beri* is readily treatable with supplemental thiamine. However, excess thiamine supplementation is typically not of benefit and does not prevent cancer. There are other examples of vitamin deficiency-related illnesses and complications that are reversed with replacement of the vitamin. However, increased doses do not necessarily translate into better health.

Phytonutrients (again, the same as phytochemicals), on the other hand, are a different story. The prefix *phyto-* refers to plants; the suffix –nutrient refers to a compound that possesses potential health benefits. As such, a phytonutrient is a chemical compound from a plant or plant by-product that has the potential to have a positive impact on health. A major difference from a vitamin, is that there are no phytonutrient deficiency diseases that are reversed with intake of the lacking phytonutrient. However, when it comes to disease prevention, phytonutrients play a major role based on accumulating published data in the medical literature.

Phytonutrients are found in fruits, vegetables, whole grains, herbs, spices, coffee, cacao beans, and tea and provide much of their colors and unique flavors. There are literally thousands of phytonutrients and a thorough discussion is beyond the aim and scope of this book. However, some salient points will be offered since these compounds are important in the prevention of various cancers. Indeed, some authors have used the term "chemoprevention" as it relates to a phytonutrient-rich diet in the prevention of cancer.[1] Johnson and colleagues published a seminal article two decades ago that examined the potential anticarcinogenic effects of various plant compounds that later became known as phytonutrients or phytochemicals.[2] Since that time, hundreds, if not thousands, of studies and publications relating to phytonutrients have emerged, giving much credence to the concept that these compounds are a valuable tool in achievement of good health. Indeed, as I write this sentence, searching the medical database Pubmed revealed 13,029 articles using the search term "phytonutrients." Searching the same term on Google revealed 1,910,000 results!

Numerous studies show an inverse relationship between a plant-based diet and cancer risk. A study published in 1992 reviewed evidence available at that time that individuals with low vegetable and fruit intake had twice the risk of developing cancer as individuals with the highest intake.[3] More studies in the 1990's and early 2000's confirmed that there was "convincing" evidence that vegetables and fruits were protective against various respiratory and digestive cancers.[4] Although there are many potential confounding reasons for this, it is very plausible that phytonutrients are largely responsible for decreasing cancer risk. This is because many of these compounds act as antioxidants that limit and/or prevent damage to cells and DNA—which ultimately culminates in cancer. Since DNA is the genetic code responsible for healthy cell function, damage to DNA can have major ill-effects on cell health, resulting in cancer.

Some phytonutrients downregulate cancer cell growth pathways which may lead to death of cancer cells, a phenomenon known as "*apoptosis.*" There are literally dozens of complicated and intertwining pathways by which cancer cells proliferate and spread (metastasize). Additionally, as cancer cells grow, they acquire more changes in their DNA and become resistant to chemotherapy and radiation treatments. This is one of the main reasons why a patient with a cancer responding to treatment experiences "relapse" or progression of their disease. Once this occurs, cancer can be very difficult to control with chemotherapy or radiation. As such, prevention of the malignant transformation of a normal cell is vital. Since phytonutrients act as antioxidants, they may prevent damage to DNA structure and subsequent gene changes that lead to cancer. Additionally, if a cell becomes cancerous, phytonutrients can inhibit growth, invasion, and metastasis of that cell. Many laboratory studies involving human cancer cell lines and rodents have shown that numerous phytochemicals from a variety of foods can inhibit cancer cell growth and lead to cell death (*apoptosis*). *Table 1* lists some of the most studied phytonutrients.

Table 1: Common phytonutrients[†]

Carotenoids

    α/β-carotenes

    Lutein

    Zeaxanthin

    Lycopene

Phenolic acids and flavonoids

    Gallic acid/vanillic/caffeic acid

    Quercetin

    Kaempferol

    Myricetin

    Apigenin

    Catechin/epicatechin /epicatechin gallate (ECG)/epigallocatechin gallate (ECGC)

    Malvidin/cyanidin

    Genistein

Organosulfur compounds

    Isothiocyanates

    Indoles

    Allylic sulfur compounds

[†]Simplified from Liu RH. J Nutr 2004;134:3480S

As noted, the anticancer effects of phytonutrients are biochemically diverse; however, a brief overview should provide the reader with an appreciation for the complexity of these fascinating nutrients.

Anticarcinogenic effects

A carcinogen is basically any chemical that, when ingested, absorbed, or inhaled, has the capacity to damage a cell's DNA and lead to malignant transformation. Some chemicals known collectively as "blocking agents" stop the activation of carcinogens or lead to excretion or inactivation of the carcinogen.[1] Detoxification and excretion of carcinogens usually occurs in the liver or intestinal tissue by an enzyme system known as *cytochrome P-450*. This system transforms toxins and carcinogens to harmless compounds that are excreted in the urine or feces. Another vital enzyme system known as *glutathione S-transferase*, acts as an antioxidant and scavenges cell-harming free radicals.

Many phytonutrients enhance or protect these enzyme systems, thereby inactivating carcinogens and keeping the cell from becoming cancerous. For example, a flavonol found in green tea known as *epigallocatechin gallate (ECG)*, has been shown to increase some of these cell-protecting enzymes.[5] Cruciferous plants such as broccoli and kale, also contain numerous antioxidants and flavonols that inhibit carcinogenesis.

Inhibition of cancer cell growth

The development and progression of cancer is an extremely complicated process and, unfortunately, despite the body's attempts at preventing a cancer cell from emerging, genetic damage invariably occurs. Once a change in DNA occurs, gene mutations follow and result in changes in cell enzyme and protein structure that alters cell growth—leading to a cell that is immortal. Cancer cells are basically cells that do not have the appropriate mechanism or machinery to "turn off" cell growth. An analogy I use with my patients is placing a large piece of duct tape over a light switch in the "on" position. The power for the light to keep shining is not turned off despite attempts to "flip" the switch off. As such, the bulb keeps burning despite attempts to turn it off. This is indeed a very simplistic analogy of what happens to a malignant cell when a growth pathway is not kept "in check" by normal cell processes. Once DNA damage occurs, cell growth cannot turn off, which is a hallmark of cancer.

Another hallmark of cancer is the inability for normal cell death to occur. Normal cells usually have a preprogrammed pathway that leads to death of the cell—a process known as *apoptosis*. If abnormal cells continue to accumulate due to lack of normal cell death (even in the absence of abnormal proliferation), a population of cancer cells accumulates leading eventually to a detectable cancer. Some cancers known as lymphomas exhibit abnormal *apoptosis* in addition to increased proliferation, which leads to accumulation of cancer cells and, eventually, symptomatic cancer.

Once genetic damage has occurred, other mutations may emerge more readily and contribute to the rapid growth and spread of a cancer. However, interruption of the growth of an established cancer cell or cells may prevent an overt cancer from developing. This is where chemoprevention through a phytonutrient-rich diet may be relevant. By daily and prolonged ("*metronomic*") ingestion of phytonutrient-rich foods, reversal of cell damage and suppression of cancer cell growth may occur. This may be through an anti-inflammatory effect, through induction of *apoptosis*, or by inhibiting various growth pathways. Many phytonutrients inhibit inflammation, which is clearly damaging to cells and can lead to cancer if it persists for a long time. Olive oil is rich in anti-inflammatory and antioxidant compounds and has been shown to decrease systemic inflammation and reduce development of several cancers.[6] *Alpha*-linolenic acid found in flaxseed is a plant-derived *omega-3*-fatty acid that has been shown to decrease inflammation through inhibition of certain enzymes such as cyclooxygenase. Decreased inflammation results in less damage to cells which limits DNA damage and cancer formation.

One of the most common and potent cancer-causing growth pathways is known as the nuclear factor *kappa beta* (NF-kB) pathway, which is found in most human malignancies. Increased activity of NF-kB results in increased cell growth and actually is a target for currently available cancer drugs such as bortezomib (Velcade®), which is used to treat a blood cancer known as multiple myeloma. A research group at the M.D. Anderson Cancer Center in Houston has described numerous spice-derived phytonutrients that inhibit the NF-kB growth pathway.[7] As noted in *Appendix 1*, notable phytonutrients that have been demonstrated to block this pathway include curcumin (found in turmeric), resveratrol (found in grapes), gingerol (found in ginger), apigenin (found in parsley and celery), and limonene (found in citrus peel).

Other cancer cell growth pathways seem to be blocked, slowed, or inhibited by diverse phytonutrients. Some of these pathways include STAT3, Hedgehog, HIF-1, PPAR, wnt-1, NRF-2 and AP-1. These pathways are exquisitely complex and scientists are only recently beginning to unfold how they cause a normal cell to become cancerous. Systemic inflammation often "turns on" some of these pathways which can lead to a rapid proliferation of the transformed cancer cell, much like a snowball rolling down a hill. Since there are numerous stimuli that may trigger a cell to become cancerous and then grow and spread, it makes intuitive sense that no one phytonutrient in isolation will decrease cancer risk. It is the "sum" of the phytonutrients ingested daily and long-term ("*metronomic*") that decreases cancer risk noted in many population based studies.[8] Additionally, preventing the development of a cancer cell or halting tumor growth while still microscopic is paramount, since as tumors grow, they acquire numerous gene mutations that activate other growth paths and render treatment less effective. This is known as the "Goldie-Coldman" hypothesis and is a fundamental concept in the science of cancer medicine. To go back to the "snowball" analogy, once the snowball reaches a critical mass, it becomes much harder to roll and takes a longer time to melt. Indeed, a small snowball can be picked up and crushed easily and it will melt quickly; not-so-much the huge snowball!

This is where the concept of *metronomic phytonutrition* may be of benefit. Since the "Seven-Countries" study was published four decades ago, it has been consistently observed that the countries surrounding the Mediterranean Sea have a lower risk of certain cancers than other parts of the globe. The evidence is pretty convincing that this lower risk is due to the DAILY and LIFELONG (e.g., consistently over time = *metronomic*) intake of fruits, vegetables, nuts, seeds, herbs, and spices (diet rich in plant-derived nutrients = phytonutrition), that provides hundreds of phytonutrients. Since carcinogenesis is a multistep process, the prolonged intake of diverse phytonutrients seems to enchance detoxification systems, scavenge free radicals, stimulate the immune system, and regulate expression of genes that control cell growth and death (*apoptosis*).[10] Over time, this may lead to suppression of the numerous growth pathways mentioned above, thus preventing the snowball from forming in the first place or stopping its growth before it becomes a huge "snowball" that cannot be stopped.

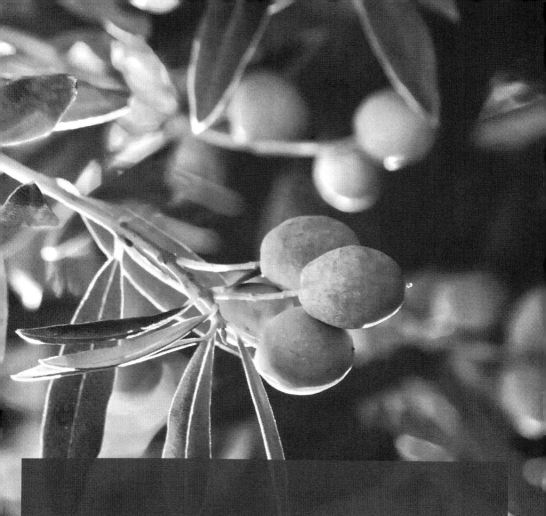

Chapter IV
Pay Attention to the Sicilians

The "Seven Countries" Study[1] popularized the term "Mediterranean Diet" and the role it plays in the prevention of coronary heart disease and cancer. This book is NOT about the Mediterranean diet specifically, but when one discusses phytonutrients, this diet takes center-stage and deserves discussion. Indeed, numerous studies that cannot be described in detail have shown that the inhabitants of the countries surrounding the Mediterranean Sea have an overall lower cancer risk compared to Western countries. These countries reside in Northern Africa (Morocco, Tunisia, and Egypt) and Europe (Spain, Italy, and Greece) as well as the Middle-East (Turkey, Israel, Syria, and Lebanon). What these culturally diverse countries share in common, is the significant consumption of phytonutrient-dense foods, namely extra-virgin olive oil, legumes, spices, vegetables, seeds, and various fruits. That being stated, India boasts very low rates of colorectal cancer—something that has been attributed to the high intake of various aromatic spices such as turmeric and cumin, amongst others.

Regions of Sicily, the largest island in the Mediterranean, contain pockets of geography that have some of the highest numbers of inhabitants over the age of 100 (centenarians). A region in the Sicani Mountains has a much higher population of centenarians (including males) than other parts of Italy, where longevity in general is not unusual. Vasto[1] and colleagues noted a 4.32-fold higher average of centenarians in this region compared to Italy as a whole. Furthermore, the female:male ratio in the Sicani region was 1.1:1, while in Italy the ratio was 4.54:1. It is well-known that females worldwide have a longer average lifespan than males; the reasons are numerous and will not be considered here. Nonetheless, this little corner of the world may have something to teach the rest of us when it comes to diet, health, and longevity.

Vasto[1] and others[2-4] have demonstrated that Centenarians and those of the "oldest-old" age group (those greater than 85 years of age) share a few things in common when it comes to diet. One of the most important is consistent and lifelong (*"metronomic"*) intake of low glycemic index (GI) foods such as whole grains, nuts, seeds, and vegetables. Foods with a low GI do not cause as abrupt and high surges in blood sugar compared to refined foods containing refined sugar, high fructose corn syrup, and white flour. The rapid rise in blood sugar causes the pancreas to release higher levels of insulin. Insulin stimulates certain cell growth factors such as insulin-like growth factor (IGF) which stimulate various pathways that can lead to cancer cell growth and metastasis.[5] While there is no conclusive proof that eating sugar "fuels" cancer in humans *per se*, a prolonged diet rich in foods with a high GI may well increase cancer risk via stimulation of IGF and growth pathways that it stimulates.

Another pattern found in the research of the oldest-old of the Mediterranean, is the consistent and essentially daily (e.g. *"metronomic"*) intake of significant amounts of extra virgin olive oil (EVOO). Extra virgin olive oil is produced by pressing the freshly picked olive fruits and collecting the oil—this is known as the "first press", which is most desirable for its health-promoting properties. Olive oil has been known to enhance health for centuries, and even King Solomon was aware of the benefits as he stated in Proverbs 21:20: "The wise store up choice food and olive oil" (Holy Bible, New International Version).

There are literally dozens of antioxidants and biochemically complex phytonutrients knowns as phenolics in EVOO. These substances (see *Appendix 1*) inhibit cell oxidation within blood vessels and block the growth of cancer cells. Oleic acid found in EVOO has been shown experimentally to decrease cellular levels of a cancer-causing gene ("oncogene") known as HER-2, which is implicated in many human cancers such as breast and stomach.[6,7] Others have shown that the Mediterranean diet rich in EVOO reduces

cancer risk.[8] For an enjoyable and educational review on olive oil, *The Seven Wonders of*

Olive Oil by Alice Alech and Cecile Le Galliard (Familius,LLC, 2017) is recommended.

Regular consumption of pizza was found to reduce the risk of digestive cancers; this may

relate to the high content of the potent antioxidant, lycopene found in tomato sauce.[9]

Diets high in *omega-6* fatty acids, from consumption of significant meat

products, tip the body's balance toward an inflammatory state. It is thought that systemic

inflammation leads to up-regulation of various cell growth pathways that can contribute

to cancer cell formation, proliferation, and spread. Increased amounts of *omega-3* fatty

acids suppress inflammation and may play a role in decreasing cancer risk. Oily fish are

an excellent source of *omega-3* fats, but flaxseed is the richest source amongst plants. By

ingesting flaxseed and fish on a frequent basis, the ratio of *omega-6* to *omega-3* decreases and

may be one of the mechanisms by which a Mediterranean-style diet reduces cancer risk.

In addition to Sicily, the other large Mediterranean island known as Crete has

a higher than average number of centenarians. One reason may be that Cretans ingest

significant amounts of EVOO and various plant foods daily, which provides constant

("*metronomic*") antioxidant effects via abundant phytonutrients and oleic acid.[10-12]

Consumption of red wine, which is abundant in phytonutrients such as resveratrol, is likely

another contributor to longevity not only in Sicily and Crete, but also throughout the

Mediterranean, especially Italy and Greece. Moderate consumption of red wine (1-2 glasses

daily) decreases the risk of cardiovascular disease by promoting a healthy lipid profile and

inducing vascular relaxation *via* release of nitric oxide. Finally, the oldest old residing in the

Mediterranean are typically non-smokers, get ample sleep, and are physically active.

The concept of "*metronomic phytonutrition*" is easily adaptable in the United States, where we are blessed with the ability to obtain high-quality foods in our supermarkets. By adjusting one's diet through incorporating combinations of spices, herbs, vegetables, fruits, seeds, nuts, whole grains, and EVOO with most meals on a daily basis and avoiding smoking, we may move a step closer to the health status of people residing in the Sicani mountains.

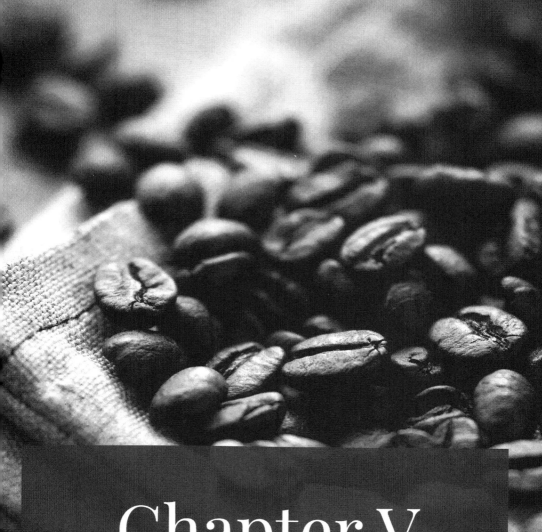

Chapter V

How Can This "*Metronomic Phytonutrition*" Concept Help?

Metronomic is a word that may be unfamiliar to many people. The word basically refers to the concept of something that is *continuous* and *regular* throughout the course of time. A metronome is a time-keeping device used by musicians to help them play their instrument in a steady and continuous fashion—"keeping the beat." *Metronomic* is a term occasionally used in the discipline of medical oncology and refers to the administration of chemotherapy on a regular or continuous basis to patients with treatment-refractory metastatic cancer.

Most of the metronomic chemotherapy regimens consist of low doses of oral drugs such as methotrexate, procarbazine, cyclophosphamide, etoposide, or capecitabine. Depending on the type of cancer, the oncologist may prescribe one drug or a combination of drugs based on studies that have shown potential benefit. Typically, a metronomic regimen consists of very low doses of the drug given every day; if side-effects occur, a few day break is suggested. Studies have shown that the continuous delivery of low-dose chemotherapy seems to inhibit the growth of blood vessels within tumors, a process known as angiogenesis.[1]

Tumors can grow to the size of about 1 millimeter without a blood supply, obtaining their nutrients from the flowing blood and surrounding tissues by diffusion. However, once a tumor mass reaches 1-2 millimeters in diameter, blood vessels need to be present within the growing mass to supply oxygen and other nutrients. Researchers have demonstrated that by giving low dose continuous therapy, the process of angiogenesis is disrupted, and tumor growth is stopped or slowed.[2] Of course, not every cancer is treated in this fashion and not every cancer responds to this type of therapy. However, some aggressive breast cancers and lymph cancers (lymphoma) may have their growth slowed or temporarily halted with this treatment approach.

How can this concept of metronomic chemotherapy be applied to human nutrition and cancer prevention? For example, the phytonutrient known as curcumin found in turmeric, has been shown in laboratory studies to inhibit angiogenesis and prevent cancer cell growth in a variety of cancers.[3-5] Curcumin has been researched for over 50 years and shown to inhibit cancer initiation, promotion, and metastasis. Curcumin can stop or slow cancer cell growth by a variety of complex mechanisms beyond the scope of this book. However, to show the reader the complexities of this phytonutrient (remember there are thousands!) a few words are worthwhile. In laboratory experiments, curcumin has been shown to impair growth of various types of cancer cells by down-regulating growth pathways (such as NF-kB, a key player in cancer growth) and decreasing various growth factors (e.g., COX-2, TNF, cyclin D1, etc.) that cause cancer cells to propogate.[6] Curcumin also is a potent antioxidant and anti-inflammatory agent.

The daily consumption of a variety of phytonutrients at most meals is thought to provide the anticancer properties of a plant-based diet. Indeed, researchers at the University of Texas M.D. Anderson Cancer Center in Houston have repeatedly shown that phytonutrients in various spices possess properties that may decrease the risk of not only cancer, but also diabetes, heart disease, autoimmune disorders, and certain neurologic problems.[6]

A significant proportion of cancers are felt to be related to diet or exposure to various environmental toxins found in cigarette smoke, sunlight, and pollution. Years of exposure to these and other toxic substances can result in systemic inflammation, which can persist for decades. Ongoing inflammation is linked to the generation of various mediators such as tumor necrosis factor (TNF), interleukins, chemokines, and other growth factors that, over time, can result in the transformation and growth of a normal cell into a cancer cell.[6,7] Suppression of this chronic inflammation may provide one avenue to decrease cancer risk. Consumption of small amounts of a variety of phytonutrients from a variety of foods exposes the body and its cells to numerous compounds that can act as antioxidants, which may prevent DNA damage, scavenge free radicals, suppress cancer cell growth pathways, and slow or stop angiogenesis. The term *"chemoprevention"* refers to the use of man-made or natural products (alone when used as drugs and in combination when ingested as food) to block or slow the development of cancer in humans.[8] The concept of *"metronomic phytonutrition"*, I believe, is an important option for safe chemoprevention: by eating a variety of plant-based foods (see *Appendix 1* for examples) at most meals every day, an individual *may* decrease his or her risk of developing cancer over their lifetime.

As previously noted, no one dietary compound can prevent cancer or any other disease, especially if it is taken in pure supplement form. The optimal action of a given phytonutrient requires the presence of other phytonutrients found in the food source and possibly other compounds present if other foods ingested concurrently. Additionally, the presence of fiber and various beneficial fats (e.g., oleic acid found in EVOO or linoleic acid found in flaxseed) may enhance absorption of phytonutrients. Consequently, taking an individual phytonutrient out of its God-given *mileau* and administered in a pill, does not result in the same beneficial effects as when ingested in whole food(s). As Aristotle stated, "the whole is greater than the sum of its parts."

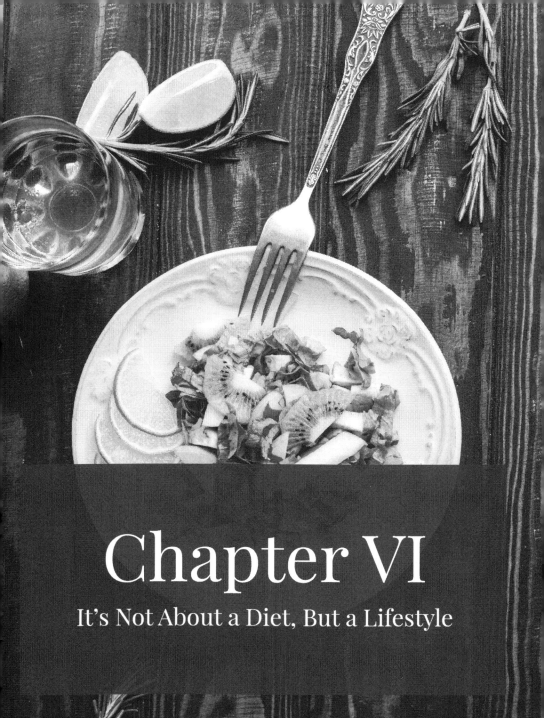

Chapter VI

It's Not About a Diet, But a Lifestyle

Generally, many would consider health as the absence of disease. Even though this is a true statement empirically, many individuals with chronic diseases (such as hypertension or high cholesterol) can be quite "healthy." Good health is more than just the absence of illness, but is also the body's ability to respond to and compensate for illness and injury as well as the subjective sense of daily well-being. Indeed, many people with a variety of chronic conditions have their sense of well-being enhanced by medication, medical procedures, avoidance of certain chemicals or toxins, exercise, and good nutritional habits. To be sure, sudden and catastrophic illness such as a ruptured aneurysm or fulminant bacterial meningitis require more than a good diet. Similarly, patients with cancer often require surgery, radiation, and/or chemotherapy for optimal treatment, whether that be curative or palliative. Nonetheless, adoption of a diet that regularly includes phytonutrients can decrease risk of some chronic diseases, as the Mediterranean diet experience has demonstrated.

"*Metronomic phytonutrition*" is about a lifetime pattern of eating—not about dieting or trying to give up this or that food or eating an apple or two a week. Yes, the Mediterranean diet is also about a lifestyle steeped in healthy plant-based eating, moderate consumption of red wine (in certain countries), daily physical activity, and rest. However, other non-Mediterranean nations have a lower risk of certain cancers due to intake of various indigenous foods and spices. As noted in a prior chapter, India boasts a very low rate of colon cancer—perhaps due to increased fiber and turmeric intake. The concept that food could improve well-being and health is also recorded in the Bible.[1] Some foods mentioned in the Bible that now have data for anticancer effects include: coriander (Exodus 16:31), olive oil (Exodus 29:2), cumin (Matthew 23:23), garlic and onion (Numbers 11:5), raisins (I Samuel 25:18), and flaxseed (Joshua 2:6), to name a few. Indeed, the New Testament supports the intake of fish (Matthew 14:17) and grains (John 6:9), which "tip the balance" more toward an anti-inflammatory state. By a reduction in systemic inflammation, cancer growth may be curtailed due to decreased production of many inflammatory cytokines which can start cancer growth or serve as fuel for growth and spread once a cell has become cancerous. The ongoing intake of phytonutrient-rich food also supplies antioxidants, glutathione, fiber, and the antioxidant vitamins C and E.[2]

Our culture is obsessed, it seems, with weight loss and leanness. There is no doubt that obesity increases risk for a host of medical problems, including cancer. For example, increased body fat leads to abnormal production of sex hormones such as estrogen, that increase the risk of breast and uterine cancers. Obesity also increases the risk of prostate cancer. However, in the absence of significant obesity, a small amount of excess body fat is not necessarily harmful. Research has shown that the glycemic index (GI, mentioned in an earlier chapter) of a given food has significant effect on one's health. Indeed, refined sugars and flour raise the blood sugar abruptly, resulting in increased insulin levels, which not only increase serum lipids, but also potentially drive tumor cell growth by increased release of various growth factors such as *IGF-1*.

Breads and cereals in moderation are *not* unhealthy, unless one has celiac sprue, an autoimmune gluten allergy. Whole grains including wheat, oats, and barley are low GI foods that avoid the sudden surge in blood sugar and tumor growth-promoting factors such as *IGF-1*. It is fairly clear that people who eat 2-3 servings of whole grains daily have a lower risk of cancers of the gastrointestinal tract and pancreas.[3] An analysis of over 40 studies revealed a 21-43% lower risk of gastrointestinal cancers with increased intake of whole grains, compared to those with scant intake.[4] Bosetti[5] and colleagues analyzed data from several studies that included 10,000 cases of cancer and 17,000 controls and reported a lower risk of airway and digestive tract cancers with increasing whole grain intake. Further, they reported that it is the type and not the presence of grain intake that increases cancer risk: refined grains such as white flour with a high GI were associated with a higher risk of cancer at several sites.[5]

In my opinion, instead of adopting a low-carbohydrate (yes, whole grains have significant carbohydrate content!) diet in an attempt to lose weight, our overall health as a population would be better off by moderate daily intake of whole grains, and not being too skinny. Whole grains contain not only fiber, but also various phenolics and antioxidants that can inhibit or slow cancer cell growth. Fiber decreases colon cancer risk by increasing stool bulk, allowing evacuation of toxic substances such as bile acids (that promote cell growth) in more rapid fashion.

There are some who caution against the daily or regular intake of olive oil, arguing that it consists of only fat and can increase bodyweight and contribute to obesity. While consumption of more than two tablespoons daily may lead to weight gain, I believe the benefits of moderate and daily ("*metronomic*") olive oil consumption outweigh any detriment, even if a person has to sacrifice weighing a few pounds more! Indeed, as *Appendix 1* demonstrates, extra virgin olive oil (EVOO) supplies numerous antioxidants, polyphenols, and healthy fats such as oleic acid, that have been demonstrated to decrease cancer risk in laboratory and epidemiologic studies. Several studies have shown that EVOO can decrease proliferation of breast cancer cells *in vitro* and in animal models. The *type* of fat, not necessarily the *presence* of fat, in the diet is what seems to be important in disease prevention. A diet enriched with EVOO compared to diets with high amounts of *omega-6* type fats such as corn oil, has been shown to slow breast cancer cell growth through a variety of mechanisms such as suppressing inflammation, decreasing oxidative stress, and enhancing the immune system's response to cancer cells.[6] Some have also shown that experimentally-induced cancers that develop in animals fed an olive oil enriched diet are less aggressive than animals not fed EVOO.[6] Olive oil may also modulate body weight and prevent obesity as compared to other fats, and this may partly explain how EVOO prevents breast and other cancers. Altogether, available data strongly supports the regular and ongoing ("*metronomic*") ingestion of EVOO in order to promote good health and possibly decrease cancer risk.

The concept of "*metronomic phytonutrition*", consequently, favors daily (or at least regular and consistent) intake of whole grains and EVOO, despite the content of carbohydrates and fat. It is the *type* of carbohydrate and fat that are important, not the mere presence, that should be considered when adopting an eating style. As long as one is not over-indulgent in caloric intake and strives for daily physical activity, it clearly is not detrimental to consume EVOO and complex carbohydrates in the form of whole grains. The addition of large amounts of fresh or frozen vegetables and fruits and various phytonutrient-rich spices and herbs on a daily basis forms the "backbone" of the "*metronomic phytonutrition*" concept, adding little fat and calories. By eating phytonutrient-dense foods at each meal, the body is exposed to the myriad of anticancer compounds almost continuously. Indeed, it is the *combination* of whole food products that likely imparts the benefit of this eating style. By ingesting a variety of phytonutrients, some of the numerous cancer growth pathways can potentially be inhibited almost continuously, thereby decreasing cancer risk. Although this is NOT proven, the evidence certainly is compelling.

There is no single "right" dietary pattern to follow with *"metronomic phytonutrition"*. Again, what is important is the daily and consistent intake of plant-based foods. Yes, there are literally hundreds of foods that are rich in phytonutrients; this is what makes a dietary pattern such as this interesting, delicious, and never boring. One can tailor their food intake to their individual taste as long as there are ample amounts of fruits and vegetables with spices such as turmeric and black pepper (along with others) in place of salt. There is *no one magic food* to be eaten that will automatically lead to good health and a life free of cancer. This is about reducing risk in a safe manner that is practical and enjoyable. The reader is referred to *Appendix 1* for an example of some of widely available phytonutrient-rich foods that can be easily incorporated into one's diet.

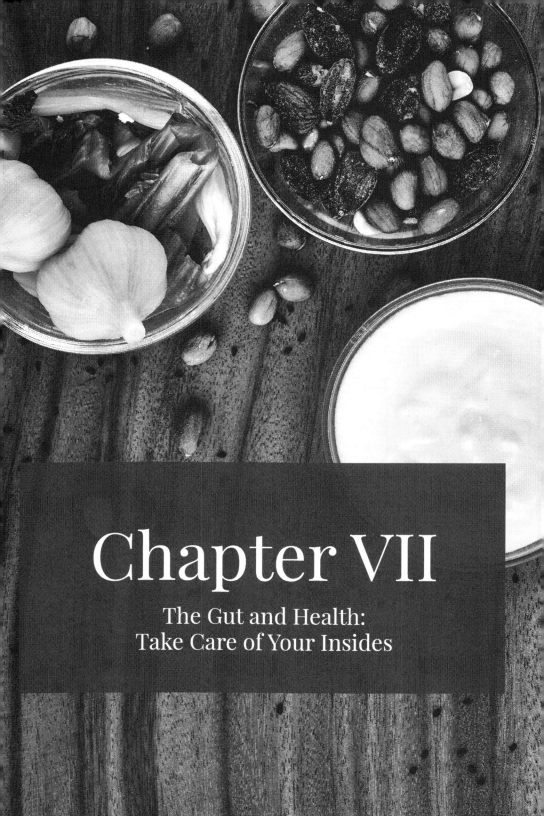

Chapter VII

The Gut and Health:
Take Care of Your Insides

The human gastrointestinal tract is a complex organ system that begins at the mouth and ends at the anus. This section is NOT meant to be a detailed discussion on the physiology of digestion (which is extremely complex), but rather intended to provide a "30,000 feet" overview of digestion, which will lead into a discussion on the emerging role that gut bacteria play in health and disease.

The salivary glands in the mouth initiate digestion by secreting amylase, an enzyme that breaks down dietary sugars. Chewing food also prepares the esophagus to transport the food into the stomach, where digestion proceeds. Through chewing and salivary gland fluids, the smaller and lubricated food bolus is further digested by stomach acids that are released by parietal cells. Parietal cells synthesize hydrochloric acid (yes, the same stuff as battery acid!) that basically breaks down stomach contents further, allowing them to pass into the first part of the small intestine—the duodenum. In the duodenum, a variety of enzymes break down sugars into more absorbable molecules for absorption across the lining of the small intestine. The pancreas releases enzymes that aid in breaking down fat and proteins (lipases and proteases, respectively). The small intestine continues for several meters as the jejunum(middle part of small intestine) and the ileum (last part of the small intestine) where nutrients such as vitamins, minerals, proteins, and many other chemicals, including phytonutrients, are absorbed and transported into the bloodstream for delivery to our cells and tissues.

At this point, the ingested food is a liquid known as "chyme", which then passes into the large intestine through the ileocecal valve, which contains a muscle that acts as a "brake" mechanism, regulating the amount of small intestinal contents that pass into the colon or large intestine. The colon is highly efficient at removing the majority of water from the liquid mixture that entered through the ileocecal valve and, by the time the mixture is eliminated, is largely solid and contains much less water. Although, absorption of water and electrolytes is a major function of the large intestine, this part of the gut plays a vital role in maintaining health and potentially promoting certain disease states.

The bacteria that live in your colon: the microbiome

The large intestine is several feet long and not only serves to absorb water and electrolytes from the intestinal contents, but also functions as a reservoir until these contents can be eliminated. It has been known for a long time, that the colon is home to numerous species of bacteria, perhaps of which the most well-known is *E.coli*. However, there are dozens of other species that reside in the colon. This population of bacteria, that numbers in the trillions,[1] consists of dozens of species of bacteria that require oxygen for growth (*aerobes*) or do not require oxygen for growth (*anaerobes*). These bacteria are first acquired when an infant descends through the mother's birth canal and becomes inhabited with bacteria from the vagina and anal area. Babies born *via Caesarean* section acquire less of their mother's favorable bacteria and are more prone to childhood ailments such as eczema and allergic disorders.[1] The population of bacteria develops over life and remains relatively constant, unless a person takes antibiotics or there is significant change in diet composition.

The majority of the time, these bacteria live out their existence peacefully with their human host. This is known as "*symbiosis*". In other words, they typically don't cause trouble while the human host provides them a place to live. However, if the population of bacteria changes with a course of antibiotics, for instance, this symbiotic relationship can be disrupted and lead to diarrhea, abdominal cramping, and inflammation. Most of the time, this is temporary and life goes on as before. However, researchers, scientists, and physicians are learning that the bacterial population living in the gut (the microbiome) is a complex interplay between the human host, the bacterial residents, and the food one eats.[1,2] This complex environment can be influenced by certain foods resulting in a favorable interaction between the bugs and the person (*symbiosis*) or an unfavorable interaction that can lead to inflammation and illness (*dysbiosis*).[3]

There is increasing evidence from scientific studies suggesting that alterations in the intestinal microbiome may be linked to over 25 disease states and/or syndromes.[4] The intestinal barrier is only one cell thick, beneath which lies nerves, blood vessels, immune cells, and lymphatic channels. Therefore, anything that changes the bacteria population into a more inflammatory/ *dysbiotic* type can disrupt this thin layer of cells.[5] This change may allow bacteria to gain access to the bloodstream, lymphatic vessels, immune system, and nervous system. In regards to the nervous system of the gut, some feel that the symptoms of irritable bowel syndrome (IBS) may be related to *dysbiotic* bacterial flora interacting with the nerves that control intestinal motility, resulting in abdominal bloating, cramps, diarrhea and/or constipation. Inflammatory bowel disease (IBD) consists of Crohn's disease and ulcerative colitis (UC), and may be linked to disruption of the intestinal microbiome leading to the inflammation characteristic of these diseases.

The basics of gut bacteria and health

The diversity of bacterial species in the human intestine is vast with significant differences in bacterial populations existing between individuals. Generally, however, certain bacterial families (*taxa*) have been associated with a positive effect on health (*symbiosis*), while others have been associated with development of certain diseases (*dysbiosis*) such as diabetes, autoimmune conditions, cardiovascular/heart disease, gastrointestinal disorders, and cancer.[1,3,6]

Prebiotics or probiotics?

Probiotics are actual live bacteria (usually *Lactobacillus* species) that can be taken in supplemental capsule form or be acquired from foods such as yogurt. Recent studies have cast doubt on whether supplementing one's diet with probiotics significantly changes the bacterial population in the human intestine and if any tangible health benefits occur. Indeed, a recent *meta-analysis* analyzed several randomized studies published over the last few years and failed to show any impact of probiotics on changing the fecal bacterial population (microbiome) in healthy adults.[7] As has been stated throughout this book, taking an individual supplement of any vitamin, mineral, phytochemical, or even bacteria, has very little reliable data to show health benefits. Indeed, it is the SUM of the diet, which includes daily and frequent (*metronomic*) ingestion of a variety of plant-based (*phytonutrition*) foods (vegetables, fruits, seeds, nuts, herbs, grains, seeds) that seems to provide the greatest health benefits.

Prebiotics are small carbohydrate (sugar) molecules found in plants that have the ability to change the composition and/or the metabolism of the gut microbiome in a beneficial way.[3] Bacterial familes such as *Bifidobacteria* and *Lactobacillus* can be increased in the intestine by consuming three common prebiotics: oligofructose, galacto-oligosaccharides, and lactulose. [5] These complex sugar molecules are found in numerous vegetables and fruits . When reaching the large intestine, prebiotics are fermented and changed into compounds by gut bacteria, called short chain fatty acids (SCFAs) that have favorable effects on the intestinal lining. Some of these beneficial effects include "tightening" the cell barrier between intestinal contents and the bloodstream, thereby preventing inflammation-producing bacteria from gaining access to the body and causing inflammation of the vessels and other organs.[1,2] It is this inflammation that is felt to contribute to coronary heart disease, heart attacks, and stroke. Another benefit of these SCFAs derived from a plant-based diet, is increased mucus production by the intestine, which also protects the bloodstream from invasion of "bad" gut bacteria and other inflammatory chemicals. One SCFA known as butyric acid, has been shown in animal studies to stimulate release of substances found in the gut wall that decrease appetite and may help one feel full earlier, leading to decreased food intake and weight loss.[18]

Studies have shown that ingesting prebiotics in the form of vegetables and fruits, can rather quickly change the microbiome to a more favorable population, which can then rapidly revert back to an unfavorable population upon changing diet back to increased animal protein and minimal plant-based foods. *Bifidobacteria* increase following ingestion of prebiotics, which is considered by some to be a good indicator of intestinal health and may improve well-being while decreasing risk of intestinal infections and allergies. Studies also suggest that increased *bifidobacteria* may have a favorable impact on diabetes and obesity, both of which lead to the number one cause of death in the Western world: cardiovascular disease. [9]

Colon cancer and the gut microbiome

Colon cancer is a common cause of cancer death. Colon cancer certainly does have a genetic component to some degree, as families with Lynch syndrome (an inherited syndrome that increases the risk of colon and other cancers) have a very high lifetime risk of colon cancer, irrespective of diet. That being stated, many colon cancers are felt to be due to the accumulation of damage to cellular DNA that leads to changes in genes that regulate cell growth and subsequent cancer development. Indeed, there is increasing evidence that many colorectal cancers can be prevented with a diet rich in plant products and low in processed meats (e.g., lunch meat, ham, etc.) and red meat/beef. This may in-part be related to nitrites found in processed meats. Nitrates are converted in the body to carcinogenic compounds known as nitrosamines.

The gut protection afforded by a plant-rich diet is quite complicated and a detailed discussion is beyond the scope of this book. However, by ingesting prebiotics, the amount of inflammation in the gut may be reduced and, over time, may limit DNA and cell damage. The gut microbiome can also directly influence growth of colon cancers, since some bacterial families (such as the *Fusobacteria* family) cause more inflammation and cell damage than others. Some studies have shown that decreased "good" bacteria such as the *Bacteroides* family and decreased bacteria that produce butyrate (which protects the intestinal cells from damage), may increase formation of colon cancers.[6,10] By ingesting a diet rich in plants (and, as a result, prebiotics), the population of bacteria switches to a less inflammatory and more protective environment, which may decrease colon tumor formation and growth.

Cardiovascular disease and your diet: It's beyond cholesterol!

For years, it has been known that diet composition is associated with risk of developing coronary heart disease—a condition in which fat-rich blockages known as plaques (e.g., *atherosclerosis*), form within the arteries on the heart surface that supply the heart muscle with blood and oxygen. If an artery becomes blocked, usually by a sudden disruption or "fracture" of a plaque, the heart muscle is robbed of bloodflow that supplies oxygen and nutrients. If this artery is not opened up or "unclogged" quickly, heart muscle is damaged (usually permanently), a condition known as a myocardial infarction (MI or "heart attack"). For many years, studies have shown that diets high in saturated animal fats (especially red meats such as beef), are linked to coronary disease and atherosclerosis. This is felt to be due to toxic fats and cholesterol which deposit in the arteries leading to plaque formation, which increases risk for not only heart attacks, but also strokes and peripheral arterial disease in the legs (PAD).

Studies have found a lower incidence of cardiovascular disease in vegetarians, the Seventh Day Adventist population (who are typically vegetarian or vegan), and those residing in the Mediterranean region, as the Seven Countries Study has shown. What these groups have in common, is the consistent, high intake of plant-based foods such as fruits, vegetables, seeds, nuts, spices, and herbs. The bulk of this book has explained how phytonutrients are beneficial to health and that populations who eat larger amounts of plants often consume less red meat, which may explain the lower risk of high cholesterol and heart disease. However, researchers are now learning that cardiovascular disease seems to go beyond cholesterol and is likely related to what lives in our large intestine.

Meat, especially red meats, eggs, liver, and pork contain significant amounts of a compound known as phosphatidylcholine, or lecithin (I will refer to this as lecithin from now on since it is easier to type and pronounce). Some have shown that diets rich in lecithin are associated with a higher risk of atherosclerosis—this is not surprising since this compound is primarily found in red meats and eggs.[11] Ingested lecithin is broken down by fat-digesting enzymes in the small intestine into a variety of choline-containing compounds such as choline, phosphocholine, and glycerophosphocholine.[11,12] These three compounds, upon reaching the large intestine and interacting with bacteria, are ultimately converted or metabolized into a chemical called *trimethylamine-N-oxide* (TMAO).[12] Studies have shown that TMAO can increase cholesterol accumulation in artery walls, which is associated with atherosclerosis, cardiovascular disease, and death.[11] Indeed, researchers have shown an increased risk of cardiovascular events (heart attacks, strokes, etc.) in people with higher blood TMAO levels, independent of traditional factors for cardiovascular disease (e.g., hypertension, high cholesterol, diabetes mellitus).[11-13]

A group of researchers published an elegant study in the *New England Journal of Medicine* showing that dietary lecithin intake increases blood TMAO levels. To demonstrate this, the researchers measured TMAO levels in blood and urine in 40 healthy participants after the ingestion of two hard-boiled eggs, which are rich in lecithin. They noted significant increases in urine and blood TMAO levels shortly after ingestion.[12] Several participants were then administered antibiotics for one week to suppress intestinal bacteria. These participants returned after antibiotic therapy and again ingested two eggs. In this group, urine and blood TMAO levels did NOT increase, suggesting that suppression of intestinal flora by the antibiotics prevented conversion of the lecithin-derived choline compounds into TMAO. One month later off antibiotics, the same protocol was repeated with a rise in TMAO levels after egg ingestion. [12] This reinforces the pivotal role that gut bacteria play in the conversion of lecithin/phosphatidylcholine into TMAO.

Studies have also shown a higher risk of cardiovascular disease in people with high blood levels of the amino acid, *L-carnitine*, which also increases TMAO levels.[13] A group of researchers from the Cleveland Clinic demonstrated that *L-carnitine* in red meat is converted into TMAO by intestinal bacteria.[14] This group showed that vegans and vegetarians produced much less TMAO after the ingestion of red meat compared to omnivores, those who ingest meat as well as plants. This finding suggests that the microbiome of vegetarians is populated with bacteria that cannot efficiently convert *L-carnitine* into toxic TMAO, compared to those who regularly ingest meat.[13,14] Regular consumption of meat and lecithin-rich foods changes the microbiome into a more toxic, or *dysbiotic*, environment that favors generation of TMAO and increases the risk of atherosclerosis and cardiovascular disease.[15] Indeed, studies have shown that vegetarians/ vegans have lower baseline TMAO blood levels compared to people who regularly consume red meat.[14]

Elevated baseline TMAO is independently associated with not only cardiovascular disease, but also diabetes, kidney disease, heart failure, and death.[1,13-15] More recent studies have shown than patients presenting to a hospital with a heart attack syndrome or chest pain and who have elevated TMAO levels, have inferior outcomes not only in the short-term, but also in the long-term compared with those with lower levels.[16,17] Also, increased TMAO levels in patients with congestive heart failure predicts a higher risk of death, even after correcting or adjusting for traditional cardiovascular risk factors (e.g., hypertension, high cholesterol, diabetes).[17] Finally, a recent study published in the *American Journal of Clinical Nutrition* showed that among 120,000 women and men participating in the longitudinal Nurses' Health Study and Health Professionials Follow-up Study, individuals in the highest quintile TMAO level had higher all-cause and cardiovascular mortality compared to those with levels in the lowest quintile; this was most marked in diabetics.[18] Altogether, this accumulating data supports the "*metronomic phytonutrition*" concept since regular, daily consumption of a plant-based diet apparently induces changes in gut microbiome that seems to decrease risk of atherosclerosis and heart disease, and possibly, colon cancer.

Notes

Chapter 1: Another nutrition book?

1.   Fortmann SP, Burda BU, Senger CA, et al. Vitamin, mineral, and multivitamin supplements for the primary prevention of cardiovascular disease and cancer: a systematic evidence review for the U.S. Preventative Services Task Force (Internet). Rockville, MD: Agency for Healthcare Research and Quality (US); 2013 Nov. Report No.: 14-05199-EF-1

2.   Lippman SM, Klein EA, Goodman PJ, et al. Effect of selenium and vitamin E on risk of prostate cancer and other cancers: the selenium and vitamin E prevention trial (SELECT). JAMA 2009;301:39-51

3.   Fortmann SP, Burda BU, Senger CA, et al. Vitamin and mineral supplements in the primary prevention of cardiovascular disease and cancer: an updated systematic evidence review for the U.S. Preventative Services Task Force. Ann Intern Med 2013;159:824-834

4.   Golden EB, Lam PY, Kardosh A, et al. Green tea polyphenols block the anticancer effects of bortezomib and other boronic acid-based proteasome inhibitors. Blood 2009;113:5927-5937

5.   Meeran SM, Katiyar SK. Cell cycle control as a basis for cancer chemoprevention through dietary agents. Front Biosci 2008;13:2191-2202

6.   Aggarwal BB, Kunnumakkara AB, Harikumar KB, et al. Potential of spice-derived phytochemicals for cancer prevention. Planta Med 2008;74:1560-1569

7.   Aggarwal BB, Shishodia S. Molecular targets of dietary agents for prevention and therapy of cancer. Biochem Pharmacol 2006;71:1397-1421

Chapter 2: Nutrition and cancer: A brief overview

1. Thygesen LC, Hvidt NC, Hansen HP, et al. Cancer incidence among Danish Seventh-day Adventists and Baptists. Cancer Epidemiol 2012;36:513-518

2. Phillips RL. Role of lifestyle and dietary habits in risk of cancer among Seventh-Day Adventists. Cancer Res 1975;35:3513-3522

3. Bamia C, Lagiou P, Buckland G, et al. Mediterranean diet and colorectal cancer risk: results from a European cohort. Eur J Epidemiol 2013;28:317-328

4. Bosetti C, Gallus S, Trichopoulou A, et al. Influence of the Mediterranean diet on the risk of cancers of the upper aerodigestive tract. Cancer Epidemiol Biomarkers Prev 2003;12:1091-1094

5. LaVecchia C, Bosetti C. Diet and cancer risk in Mediterranean countries: open issues. Public Health Nutr 2006;9:1077-1082

6. Fernandez E, Gallus S, LaVecchia C. Nutrition and cancer risk: an overview. J Br Menopause Soc 2006;12:139-142

7. LaVecchia C, Tavani A. Fruit and vegetables and human cancer. Eur J Cancer Prev 1998;7:3-8

8. Tavani A, LaVecchia C. Fruit and vegetable consumption and cancer risk in a Mediterranean population. Am J Clin Nutr 1995;61:1374S-1377S

9. Trichopoulou A, Costacou T, Bamia C, et al. Adherence to a Mediterranean diet and survival in a Greek populatin. N Engl J Med 2003;348:2599-2608

Chapter 3: What are phytonutrients?

1. Johnson IT. Phytochemicals and cancer. Proc Nutr Soc 2007;66:207-215

2. Johnson I, Williamson G, Musk S. Nutr Res Rev 1994;7:175-204

3. Block G, Patterson B, Subar A. Fruit, vegetables, and cancer prevention: a review of the epidemiologic evidence. Nutr Cancer 1992;18:1-29

4. Steinmetz KA, Potter JD. Vegetables, fruit, and cancer prevention: a review. J Am Diet Assoc 1996;96:1027-1039

5. Chou FP, Chu YC, Hsu JD, et al. Specific induction of glutathione S-transferase GSTM2 subunit expression by epigallocatechin gallate in rat liver. Biochem Pharmacol 2000;60:643-650

6. Owen RW, Haubner R, Wurtele G, et al. Olives and olive oil in cancer prevention. Eur J Cancer Prev 2004;13:319-326

7. Sung B, Prasad S, Yadav VR, et al. Cancer and diet: how are they related? Free Radical Res 2011;45:864-879

8. Sofi F, Cesari F, Abbate R, et al. Adherence to Mediterranean diet and health status: meta-analysis. BMJ 2008;337:a1344.doi:10.1136/bmj.a1344

9. Keys A. Seven countries: a multivariate analysis of death and coronary heart disease. Cambridge, MA: Harvard University Press, 1980

10. Liu RH. Health benefits of fruit and vegetables are from additive and synergistic combinations of phytochemicals. Am J Clin Nutr 2003;78:517S-520S

Chapter 4: Pay attention to the Sicilians

1. Vasto S, Rizzo C, Caruso C. Centenarians and diet: what they eat in the Western part of Sicily. Immunity Aging 2012;9:10-16

2. Poulain M, Pes GM, Grasland C, et al. Identification of a geographic area characterized by extreme longevity in the Sardinia island: the AKEA study. Exp Gerontol 2004;39:1423-1429

3. Caselli G, Lipsi RM. Survival differences among the oldest old in Sardinia: who, what, where, and why? Demograph Res 2006;14:267-294

4. Lio D, Malaguarnera M, Maugeri D, et al. Laboratory parameters in centenarians of Italian ancestry. Exp Gerontol 2008;43:119-122

5. Macaulay VM. Insulin-like growth factors and cancer. Br J Cancer 1992;65:388-392

6. Menendez JA, Lupu R. Mediterranean dietary traditions for the molecular treatment of human cancer: anti-oncogenic actions of the main olive oils monounsaturated fatty acid oleic acid (18:1n-9). Curr Pharmaceut Biotech 2013;14:495-502

7. Colomer R, Menendez JA. Mediterranean diet, olive oil, and cancer. Clin Transl Oncol 2006;8:15-21

8. LaVecchia C. Mediterranean diet and cancer. Public Health Nutr 2004;7:965-968

9. Gallus S, Bosetti C, LaVecchia C. Mediterranean diet and cancer risk. Eur J Cancer Prev 2004;13:447-452

10. Trichopouloua A, Dilis V. Olive oil and longevity. Mol Nutr Food Res 2007;51:1275-1278

11. Trichopoulou A, Vasilopoulou E. Mediterranean diet and longevity. Br J Nutr 2000;84:205S-209S

12. Trichopouloua A, Critselis E. Mediterranean diet and longevity. Eur J Cancer Prev 2004;13:453-456

Chapter 5: How can this *"metronomic phytonutrition"* concept help?

1. Lien K, Georgsdottir S, Sivanthian L, et al. Low-dose metronomic chemotherapy: a systematic literature analysis. Eur J Cancer 2013;49:3387-3395

2. Merritt WM, Danes CG, Shahzad MM, et al. Anti-angiogenic properties of metronomic topotecan in ovarian carcinoma. Cancer Biol Ther 2009;8:1596-1603

3.	Stan SD. Chemoprevention strategies for pancreatic cancer. Nat Rev Gastroenterol Hepatol 2010;7:347-356

4.	Wilken R, Veena MS, Wang MB, et al. Curcumin: a review of anticancer properties and therapeutic activity in head and neck cancer. Mol Cancer 2011;10:12. Doi 10:.1186/1476-4598-10-12.

5.	LoTempio MM, Veena MS, Steele HL, et al. Curcumin suppresses growth of head and neck squamous cell carcinoma. Clin Cancer Res 2005;11:6994-7002

6.	Aggarwal BB, Kunnumakkara AB, Harikumar KB, et al. Potential of spice-derived phytochemicals for cancer prevention. Planta Med 2008;74:1560-1569

7.	Aggarwal BB, Shishodia S, Sandur SK, et al. Inflammation and cancer : how hot is the link? Biochem Pharmacol 2006;72:1605-1621

8.	Ganguly C. Flavoring agents used in Indian Cooking and their anticarcinogenic properties. Asian Pacific J Cancer Prev 2010;11:25-28

Chapter 6: It's not about a diet, but a lifestyle

1.	Berry EM, Arnoni Y, Aviram M. The Middle Eastern and Biblical origins of the Mediterranean diet. Public Health Nutr 2011;14:2288-2295

2.	Simopoulos AP. The Mediterranean diets: what is so special about the diet of Greece? The scientific evidence. J Nutr 2001;131:3065S-3073S

3.	Gil A, Ortega RM, Maldonado J. Wholegrain cereals and bread: a duet of the Mediterranean diet for the prevention of chronic diseases. Public Health Nutr 2011;14:2316-2322

4.	Slavin J. Whole grains and human health. Nutr Res 2004;17:99-110

5.	Bosetti C, Pelucchi C, LaVecchia C. Diet and cancer in Mediterranean countries: carbohydrates and fats. Public Health Nutr 2009;12:1595-1600

6.	Escrich E, Moral R, Solanas M. Olive oil, an essential component of the Mediterranean diet, and breast cancer. Public Health Nutr 2011;14:2323-2332

Chapter 7: The gut and health: Take care of your insides

1. Hansen TH, Gobel RJ, Hansen T, et al. The gut microbiome in cardiometabolic health. Genome Med 2015;7:33-49

2. Schroeder BO, Bäckhed F. Signals from the gut microbiota to distant organs in physiology and disease. Nat Med 2016;22:1079-1089

3. Roberfroid M, Gibson GR, Hoyles L, et al. Prebiotic effects: metabolic and health benefits. Br J Nutr 2010;104:S1-S63

4. de Vos WM, de Vos EAJ. Role of intestinal microbiome in health and disease: from correlation to causation. Nutr Rev 2012;70:455-565

5. Bosscher D, Breynaert A, Pieters L, et al. Food-based strategies to modulate the composition of the intestinal microbiota and their associated health effects. J Physiol Pharmacol 2009;60:5S-11S

6. Zackular JP, Baxter NT, Iverson KD, et al. The gut microbiome modulates colon tumorigenesis. M Bio 2013;4:e00692-00713

7. Kristenson NB, Bryup T, Allin KH, et al. Alterations in fecal microbiota composition by probiotic supplementation in healthy adults: a systemic review of randomized controlled trials. Genome Med 2016;8:52-63

8. Tolhurst G, Heffron H, Lam YS, et al. Short-chain fatty acids stimulate glucagon-like peptide-1 secretion via the G-protein-coupler receptor FFAR2. Diabetes 2012;61;364-371

9. Macfarlane S, Macfarlane GT, Cummings JH. Review article: prebiotics in the gastrointestinal tract. Aliment Pharmacol Ther 2006;24:701-714

10. Tözün N, Vardareli E. Gut microbiome and gastrointestinal cancer: les liaisons dangereuses. J Clin Gastroenterol 2016;50:1915-1965

11. Wang Z, Klipfell E, Bennett BJ, et al. Gut flora metabolism of phosphatidylcholine promotes cardiovascular disease. Nature 2011;472:57-63

12. Tang WHW, Wang Z, Levison BS, et al. Intestinal microbial metabolism of phosphatidylcholine and cardiovascular risk. N Engl J Med 2013;368:1575-1584

13. Koeth RA, Wang Z, Levison BS, et al. Intestinal microbiota metabolism of L-carnitine, a nutrient in red meat, promotes atherosclerosis. Nat Med 2013;19:576-585

14. Lynch SV, Pedersen O. The human intestinal microbiome in health and disease. N Engl J Med 2016;375:2369-2379

15. Suzuki T, Heaney LM, Jones DJ, et al. Trimethylamine N-oxide and risk stratification after acute myocardial infarction. Clin Chem 2017;63:420-428

16. Li XS, Obeid S, Klingenberg R, et al. Gut microbiota-dependent trimethylamine N-oxide in acute coronary syndromes: a prognostic marker for incident cardiovascular events beyond traditional risk factors. Eur Heart J 2017; 38:814-824

17. Suzuki T, Heaney LM, Bhandari SS, et al. Trimethylamine N-oxide and prognosis in acute heart failure. Heart 2016;102:841-848

18. Zheng Y, Li Y, Rimm EB, et al. Dietary phosphatidylcholine and risk of all-cause and cardiovascular-specific mortality among US women and men. Am J Clin Nutr 2016;104:173-180

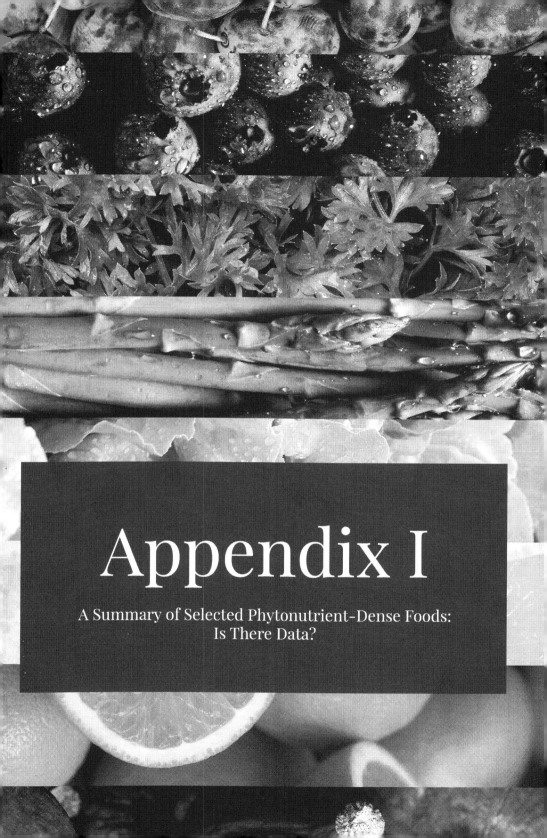

Appendix I

A Summary of Selected Phytonutrient-Dense Foods:
Is There Data?

There are literally thousands of phytonutrients found in numerous foods worldwide. However, one does not need to travel the globe in search of phytonutrient-rich foods! This section presents a selected summary of widely-available foods that should be easy to incorporate into one's daily diet. This listing is by no means exhaustive and authoritative, but rather, offers the reader a "starting point" for adopting the lifestyle of eating phytonutrient-rich foods. I chose many of the foods based on my own cooking experience, personal study of the Mediterreanean diet, and reviewing studies from the medical literature. I have provided a brief introduction on each food followed by a short discussion on anticancer properties based on studies published in the medical literature. As a physician, assessing data is vital when making not only medical recommendations, but also when counseling people on dietary changes they should consider. Again, there is no guarantee that eating any of these foods will stop cancer or any disease from developing. That being stated, however, there is fairly compelling data (as the reader will soon see) that incorporation of phytonutrients into one's diet as part of a healthy lifestyle (one that includes physical activity and avoidance of smoking and dietary excesses!) may reap potential benefit when it comes to reducing risk of not only cancer, but also cardiovascular and inflammatory diseases.

List of Phytonutrient-Dense Foods

Almonds	74	Garlic	116
Apples	76	Ginger	118
Basil	78	Grapes	120
Black Beans	80	Green Tea	122
Black Pepper	82	Kale	124
Blueberries	84	Lentils	126
Caraway Seed	86	Maple Syrup	128
Carrot	88	Mustard Seed	130
Celery	90	Olive Oil	132
Cherry	92	Onions	134
Chickpeas	94	Oregano	136
Chili Peppers	96	Parsley	138
Citrus Peel	98	Pomegranate	140
Cocoa	100	Quinoa	142
Coffee	102	Rosemary	144
Coriander	104	Sunflower Seeds	146
Cranberries	106	Tomato Paste	148
Cumin Seed	108	Turmeric	150
Dates	110	Vanilla	152
Fennel Seed	112	Walnuts	154
Flaxseed	114		

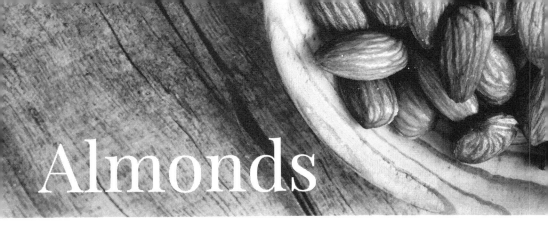

Almonds

Background

  The almond is considered a tree nut that belongs to the genus *Prunus*. The fruit of the almond tree is known as a drupe and consists of an outer hull surrounding a hard shell which contains the edible seed. The almond is actually not a true nut and belongs to the same genus as the peach. The almond is native to the Mediterranean but is widely grown in warmer parts of Europe and the United States, which is the world's leading supplier. Almonds are versatile and may be eaten raw or roasted, whole or slivered, or even ground into a flour-like meal.

Anticancer properties

  Almonds are rich in the antioxidant vitamin E, which may prevent cellular damage, as well as dietary fiber, which decreases colon cancer risk by increasing stool bulk and fecal transit. A variety of phytonutrients are found in almonds such as caretenoids, phenolic acids, flavonoids, and proanthocyanidins, which possess anti-inflammatory, antiproliferative, and antioxidant properties. It is well-established that chronic systemic inflammation increases cancer risk and that almonds have been shown to quell inflammation *via* their phytonutrient and fatty acid profile. Davis and colleagues noted that rats injected with a carcinogen to promote colon cancer were less likely to develop cell damage if they were fed an almond-rich diet compared to those animals fed a control diet; these authors suggested that almond consumption may reduce colon cancer risk. Observational population-based studies have noted an inverse association between tree nut intake, such as almonds, and cancer in general.

Bibliography

- Bolling BW, Chen CY, McKay DL, et al. Tree nut phytochemicals: composition, antioxidant activity, bioactivity, impact factors. A systemic review of almonds, Brazil nuts, cashews, hazelnuts, macadamias, pecans, pine nuts, pistachios, and walnuts. Nutr Res Rev 2011;24:244-275

- Chen CY, Blumberg JB. Phytochemical composition of nuts. Asian Pac J Clin Nutr 2008;17:329S-332S

- Davis PA, Iwahashi CK. Whole almonds and almond fractions reduce aberrant crypt foci in a rat model of colon carcinogenesis. Cancer Lett 2001;165:27-33

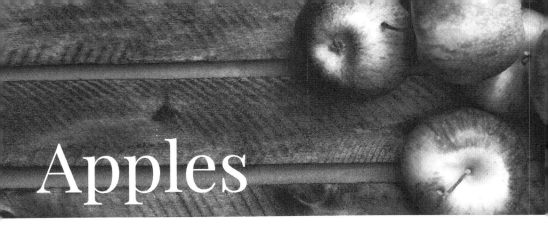

Apples

Background

The apple, *Malus* species, is perhaps one the most well-known and consumed foods in modern culture. The health benefits of the apple have been appreciated for many years and most people are familiar with the adage "an apple a day keeps the doctor away." Apples are ubiquitous in the United States and, unlike many other fruits, keep well for many months in cold storage making them available throughout the year.

Anticancer properties

Evidence suggests that apples may prevent several cancers through the action of several phytonutrients present in the flesh, but mainly in the peel. The apple contains numerous phytonutrients, with flavonoids and phenolic acids constituting the majority. Apples are the largest source of phenolics supplied in the American diet. Quercetin is a flavonoid that possesses significant antioxidant activity. Antioxidants scavenge and consume free-radicals (such as hydroxyl radical, -OH, and hydrogen peroxide, H_2O_2) that damage DNA, which may lead to cancer. Quercetin also decreases cell growth, tumor blood vessel growth (angiogenesis), and inflammation, all of which are associated with cancer development. Quercetin has slowed carcinogen-induced cancer growth in laboratory rodents.

Liver, colon, and prostate cancer cells are inhibited *in vitro* by apple peel extract, which contains not only quercetin, but other phtyonutrients such as procyanidins, catechins, triterpenoids, gallic acid, chlorogenic acid, and phloridzin. Quercetin has been shown to inhibit or block a tumor gene known as *p53* in breast cancer cells. Chlorogenic acid is an important free-radical scavenger that is found in higher concentration in apple peels compared to the flesh. Anthocyanins are another group of antioxidants which are responsible for imparting red, blue, and purple colors to various fruits and vegetables. Rome and Red Delicious varieties possess the highest level of antioxidants at least in part due to the high anthocyanin content present in the peel. Anthocyanins inhibit cell growth through various mechanisms.

Population-based studies suggest that apples may modestly decrease the risk of a variety of cancers. Consumption of at least one apple daily has been show to decrease risk of cancers of the esophagus, colon, mouth, throat, breast, ovary, kidney, and prostate by 10-20% in various studies. Gallus and colleagues found that the decreased cancer risk with apple consumption was independent of smoking, weight, other fruit consumption, alcohol intake, and exercise.

Bibliography

- Boyer J, Liu RH. Apple phytochemicals and their health benefits. Nutr J 2004;3:5-20.

- Gallus S, Talamini R, Giacosa A, et al. Does an apple a day keep the oncologist away? Ann Oncol 2005;16:1841-1844

- Hung H. Dietary quercetin inhibits proliferation of lung carcinoma cells. Forum Nutr 2007;60:146-157

- Lee KW, Kim YJ, Kim DO, et al. Major phenolics in apple and their contribution to the total antioxidant capacity. J Agric Food Chem. 2003;51:6516-6520.

- Murakami A, Ashida H, Terao J. Multitargeted cancer prevention by quercetin. Cancer Lett 2008;269:315-325

- Wolfe K, Wu X, Liu RH. Antioxidant activity of apple peels. J Agric Food Chem 2003;51:609-614

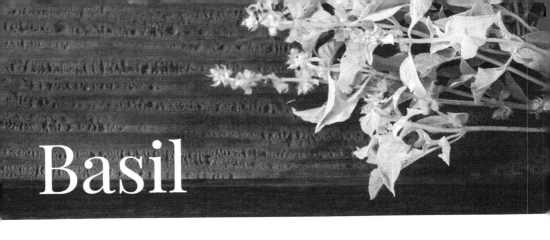

Basil

Background

Basil (*Ocimum basilicum*) is a leafy aromatic plant grown worldwide not only for its characteristic flavor, but also for its medicinal properties. Basil leaf can be used dried or fresh, but is perhaps most recognized when mixed with olive oil, cheese, and pine nuts to make pesto. The genus has many species, but is widely available and recently has been shown to possibly decrease cancer risk.

Anticancer properties

Leaf extract of basil has been shown to exhibit significant antioxidant capabilities in mice by increasing liver levels of potent antioxidants such as glutathione reductase, superoxide dismutase, and catalase. These enzymes detoxify a variety of carcinogens and toxins as they pass through the liver and other organs. Essential oils from basil were toxic to human cervical and larynx cancer cell lines in separate studies. Basil leaf extract reduced the size of melanoma tumors and increased survival in rodents. A recently published study by Shimizu and colleagues demonstrated that extracts of one species of basil leaf inhibited growth, spread, invasion, and increased *apoptosis* (cell death) of pancreatic cancer cells *in vitro*. The same researchers showed that injections of basil leaf extract into mice with pancreas cancer affected genes that decreased metastasis and increased *apoptosis*.

Bibliography

- Dasgupta T, Rao AR, Yadava PK. Chemoodulatory efficacy of basil leaf (*Ocimum basilicum*) on drug metabolizing and antioxidant enzymes, and on carcinogen-induced skin and forestomach papillomagenesis. Phytomedicine 2004;11:139-151

- Kathirvel P, Ravi S. Chemical composition of the essential oil from basil (*Ocimum basilcium Linn.*) and its *in vitro* cytotoxicity against HeLa and HEp-2 human cancer cell lines and NIH 3T3 mouse embryonic fibroblasts. Nat Prod Res 2012;26:1112-1118

- Monga J, Sharma M, Tailor N, et al. Antimelanoma and radioprotective activity of alcoholic aqueous extract of different species of Ocimum in C(57)BL mice. Pharm Biol 2011;49:428-436

- Shimizu T, Torres MP, Chakraborty S, et al. Holy Basil leaf extract decreases tumorigenicity and metastasis of aggressive human pancreatic cancer cells *in vitro* and *in vivo*: potential role in therapy. Cancer Lett 2013;336:270-280

Black Beans

Background

Black beans (*Phaselous vulgaris*) are members of the legume family and are utilized in a variety of cultures due to their excellent protein and fiber load and relatively low cost. The black bean and other dried beans, are a staple in African, Asia, Mexico, South America, Cuba, and Central America. Black beans are versatile and can be purchased in dried or canned form. Due to their high fiber and antioxidant content, black beans are gaining recognition in their ability to decrease the risk of chronic illnesses such as cardiovascular disease, diabetes, and cancer.

Anticancer properties

Similar to chick pea, black beans contain large amounts of fiber which is converted into the short chain fatty acid (SCFA), butyrate, which inhibits carcinogenesis within colonic cells. The dark skin of black beans contains a variety of phytochemical antioxidants such as triterpenoids and flavonoids that decrease oxidative stress in many cells, especially the gastrointestinal tract. The anthocyanins delphindin, petunidin, and malvidin impart the black hue to the seed coat of the black bean. Kaempferol and quercetin are flavonoids that possess antioxidant properties that decrease cellular stresses and scavenge free radicals that cause DNA damage — important steps in the formation of cancer. Extracts of black bean seed coats inhibited proliferation of several cancer cell lines. Other experimental data suggest that saponins may decrease the risk of colon and liver cancer in animals and that genistein (an isoflavone found in soy beans) inhibited *in vitro* growth of breast cancer cells.

A decreased incidence of colon cancer in humans has been observed with higher intake of insoluble fiber that beans provide; this is in-part due to the anticancer effect of butyrate on the colonic epithelium. Animal studies suggest that black beans may decrease the risk of liver and breast cancer in animals, although data in humans is lacking. An epidemiological study suggested that higher bean intake in general was associated with a lower risk of acute myeloid leukemia.

Bibliography

- Dong M, He X, Liu RH. Phytochemicals of black bean seed coats: isolation structure elucidation, and their antiproliferative and antioxidative activities. J Agric Food Chem 2007;55:6044-6051

- Guajardo-Flores D, Serna-Saldivar SO, Gutierrez-Uribe JA. Evaluation of the antioxidant and antiproliferative activities of extracted saponins and flavonols from germinated black beans. Food Chem 2013;141:1497-1503

- Yamamura Y, Oum R, Gbito KY, et al. Dietary intake of vegetables, fruits, and meat/beans as potential risk factors of acute myeloid leukemia: a Texas case-control study. Nutr Cancer 2013;65:1132-1140

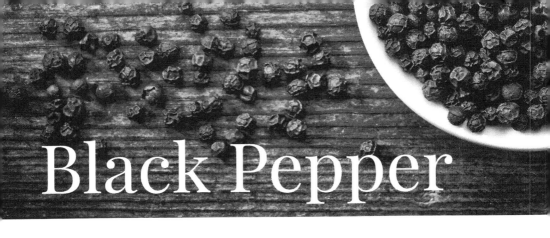

Black Pepper

Background

Black pepper (*Piper nigrum*) is a flowering vine which produces berries that are dried and used worldwide as an aromatic spice. Pepper is widely used in homes and restaurants in the United States and, despite being so taken for granted, possesses significant health-promoting properties. Black pepper is native to India, although Vietnam is currently the largest exporter. Pepper has played an important part in the world economy being used as money in some ancient cultures and medicine in other cultures.

Anticancer properties

Black pepper contains many extractable compounds including various terpenes and perhaps the most important anticancer compound, piperine. Piperine is an antioxidant responsible for the pungent aroma and spicy taste of black pepper and increases the absorption of curcumin, a potent anticancer compound found in turmeric. Piperine has been demonstrated *in vitro* to decrease reactive oxygen species, quench free radicals, and inhibit lipid peroxidation, all of which lead to cell membrane damage and contribute to cancer cell transformation. Piperine inhibits proliferation and increases *apoptosis* of some breast, rectal, and prostate cancer cell lines and blocks various signaling pathways important for cancer growth. Piperine has been shown to inhibit angiogenesis, the formation of new blood vessels that support tumor growth. Altogether, research is demonstrating that black pepper may prevent a variety of human cancers.

Bibliography

- Do MT, Kim HG, Khanal T, et al. Antitumor efficacy of piperine in the treatment of human HER2-overexpressing breast cancer cells. Food Chem 2013;141:2591-2599

- Samykutty A, Shetty AV, Dakshinamoorthy G, et al. Piperine, an bioactive component of pepper spice exerts therapeutic effects on androgen dependent and androgen independent prostate cancer cells. PLoS One 2013;8:e65889

- Srinivasan K. Black pepper and its pungent principle-piperine: a review of diverse physiological effects. Crit Rev Food Sci Nutr 2007;47:735-748

- Yaffe PB, Doucette CD, Walsh M, et al. Piperine impairs cell cycle progression and causes reactive oxygen species-dependent *apoptosis* in rectal cancer cells. Exp Mol Pathol 2013;94:109-114

Blueberries

Background

Blueberries (*Vaccinium angustifolium,* or wild blueberry, and *Vaccinium corymbosum*, or cultivated blueberry) are found throughout North America and have been heralded as one of the most antioxidant-rich foods that may decrease the risk of several chronic diseases, including cancer. Blueberries are most abundant in late spring and early summer. Wild blueberries are typically smaller and sweeter than farm-raised (cultivated) blueberries, which may be twice the size of the wild-grown type.

Anticancer properties

Although blueberries contain numerous phytonutrients, it is the compounds that impart the beautiful blue color which are the most beneficial with regards to cancer prevention: anthocyanins. Anthocyanins are found in a variety of fruits and vegetables and are responsible for the intense red, blue, and purple hues of apples, blueberries, and cabbage, respectively. Anthocyanins are potent antioxidants, possessing the ability to scavenge and dispose of free-radicals, potentially preventing DNA damage. Additionally, anthocyanins prevent and/or slow the growth of cancer cells as well as lead to death of cancer cells, (*apoptosis*). Anthocyanins have been shown in laboratory experiments to stop the ability of cancer cells from spreading by blocking a protein known as matrix metalloproteinase, a compound that degrades tissues surrounding tumor cells allowing them to spread. Blueberry anthocyanins decrease the growth of colon, prostate, liver, melanoma, and breast cancer cells in laboratory *in vitro* and animal models.

Blueberries contain other compounds that possess anticancer activity such as chlorogenic acid, quercetin, petunidin, malvidin, cyanidin, triterpenoids, and ursolic acid. Ursolic acid is a phytochemical that has been shown to decrease leukemia cell growth in laboratory experiments. Resveratrol is a potent antioxidant found in dark grapes, red wine, and blueberries. Compounds similar to resveratrol called stilbenes inhibit growth of melanoma and colon cancer cells in rodents.

Anthocyanins administered in the form of black raspberry powder, were shown to decrease cell growth and increase cell death in 25 patients with colon cancer who were given this agent before surgery. Biopsies of the colon tumors were taken before and after administration of the anthocyanin supplement which showed damage to colon cancer cells but not normal cells, suggesting that anthocyanins may slow the growth of colon cancer in humans. Since anthocyanins are also found in high amounts in blueberries, it remains plausible that blueberries may prevent colon cancer; further research is needed to confirm this.

Bibliography

- Neto CC. Cranberry and blueberry: evidence for protective effects against cancer and vascular diseases. Mol Nutr and Food Res 2007;51:652-664

- Rimando AM, Kalt W, Magee JB, et al. Resveratrol, pterostilbene, and piceatannol in *Vaccinium* berries. J Agric Food Chem 2004;52:4713-4719

- Seeram NP. Berry fruits for cancer prevention: current status and future prospects. J Agric Food Chem 2008;56:630-635

- Suh N, Paul S, Hao X, et al. Pterosilbene, an active constituent of blueberries, suppresses aberrant crypt foci in the azoxymethane-induced colon carcinogenesis model in rats. Clin Cancer Res 2007;13:350-355

- Wang LS, Stoner GD. Anthocyanins and their role in cancer prevention. Cancer Lett 2008;269:281-290

- Wang LS, Sardo C, Rocha CM, et al. Effect of freeze-dried black raspberries on human colorectal cancer lesions. AACR Special Conference in Cancer Research, Advances in Colon Cancer Research. 2007, #B31

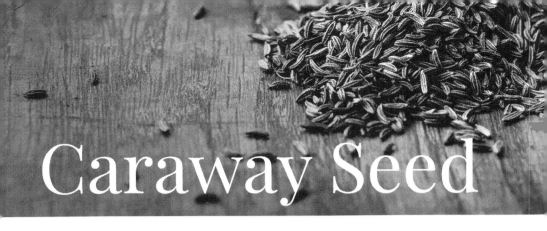

Caraway Seed

Background

Caraway (*Carum carvi*) is a plant with carrot-like leaves that is widely grown in Asia, Northern Africa, and parts of Europe. The seed is actually a fruit and grows atop long stems that first produce flowers. The aromatic aroma of caraway is derived mainly from the oils limonene and carvone, and is utilized as a breath freshener in some cultures as well as an ingredient for perfumes and soaps. Caraway has a long history of being used medicinally for a variety of ailments including diarrhea, upset stomach, flatulence, and bloating.

Anticancer properties

Caraway seed contains a variety of phytochemicals including carvone, limonene, linalool, pinen, efurfurol, carveol, and cuminic aldehyde, which contribute to the pungent aroma and antioxidant characteristics. Carvone is a volatile oil compound known as a monoterpene and has been demonstrated to act as an antioxidant *in vitro* and inhibit the formation of gastric cancer in rodents. Several flavonoids such as carotene, zea-xanthin, and carotene are also present in caraway. Caraway extract quenches hydroxyl radicals and peroxides in laboratory experiments and decreased colon cancer growth in rats. In addition, caraway extracts have decreased growth of human leukemia and *HeLa* cell lines.

Bibliography

- Allameh A, Dadkhah A, Rahbarizadeh F, et al. Effect of dietary caraway essential oils on expression of B-cantenin during 1,2-dimethylhydrazine-induced colon carcinogenesis. J Nat Med 2013;67:690-697

- Dadkhah A, Allameh A, Khalafi H, et al. Inhibitory effects of dietary caraway essential oils on 1,2 dimethylhydrazine-induced colon carcinogenesis is mediated by liver xenobiotic metabolizing enzymes. Nutr Cancer 2011;63:46-54

- Johri RK. *Cuminum cyminum* and *carvum carvi*: an update. Pharmacogn Rev 2011;5:63-72

- Kamaleeswari M, Nalini N. Dose response efficacy of caraway (*Carum carvi L.*) on tissue lipid peroxidation and antioxidant profile in rate colon carcinogenesis. J Pharm Pharmacol 2006;58:1121-113

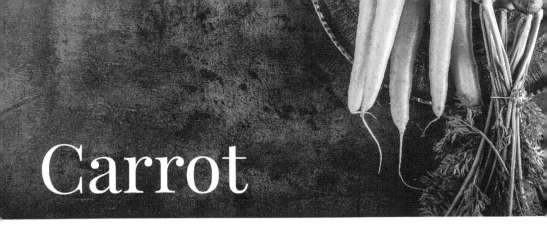

Carrot

Background

The carrot (*Daucua carota*) is a popular root vegetable, typically orange in color, although yellow, purple, red, and white varieties exist. The modern carrot likely originated in Afghanistan about 1000 years ago. Popularity spread throughout Europe, the Middle East, and India and eventually was introduced to early America by European settlers in the 17th century. Carrots are grown worldwide, but China is a leading grower. Carrots are utilized in many cuisines and are often eaten raw or cooked in a variety of ways.

Anticancer properties

Beta-carotene imparts the orange hue which contributes significant antioxidant properties and is converted in the body to vitamin A. Numerous phytochemicals known as polyacetylenes are found in carrots. Falcarindiol is a polyacetylene that is responsible for the bitter taste. Carrots contain numerous antioxidants which may protect cells from free-radical damage, which can result in cancer due to damage of DNA. Wild carrot oil has been shown to increase death (*apoptosis*) and decrease proliferation of human colon and breast cancer cells *in vitro*. Epidemiologic data suggest that regular carrot consumption may decrease the risk of bladder cancer and head and neck cancer. Fresh carrot juice administered to female breast cancer survivors resulted in increased plasma beta-carotene levels and decreased oxidative stress.

Bibliography

- Butalla AC, Crane TE, Patil B, et al. Effects of a carrot juice intervention on plasma carotenoids, oxidative stress and inflammation in overweight breast cancer survivors. Nutr Cancer 2012;64:331-341

- Freedman ND, Park Y, Subar AF, et al. Fruit and vegetable intake and head and neck cancer risk in a large United States prospective cohort study. Int J Cancer 2008;122:2330-2336

- Shebaby WN, El-Sibai M, Smith KB, et al. The antioxidant and anticancer effects of wild carrot oil extract. Phytother Res 2013;27:737-744

- Silberstein JL, Parsons JK. Evidence based principles of bladder cancer and diet. Urology. 2010;75:340-346

- Tan KW, Killeen DP, Li Y, et al. Dietary polyacetlyenes of the falcarinol type are inhibitors of breast cancer resistance protein (BRCP/ABCG2). Eur J Pharmacol 2014; 723:346-352

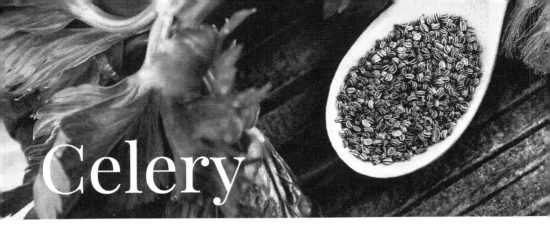

Celery

Background

Celery (*Apium graveolens*) is a widely cultivated plant with many varieties. The Pascal variety is the predominant cultivar grown in the United States. This plant has a long history, with celery leaves found in King Tut's tomb. Celery is utilized in a variety of dishes but is most often consumed raw, in a salad, or crudite trays. The plant is grown from very small seeds, which possess a variety of phytonutrients. The seed also contains a variety of volatile oils that are utilized in the perfume industry.

Anticancer properties

Celery and its seeds possess an array of phytonutrients that may prevent cancer. The characteristic aroma of fresh celery emanates from a group of compounds known as polyacetylenes. Celery seed contains several compounds that possess antioxidant and antiproliferative properties such as petroselenic acid, selinene, limonene, sedanolide, and phthalides. Some of these phytonutrients have been shown in laboratory animals to stimulate production of a detoxifying enzyme known as glutathione S-transferase. Both sedanolide and phthalides have been shown to suppress stomach cancer growth in mice. In addition, the flavonoid, apigenin, decreased gastric cancer growth in rodents. Celery seed extract increased *apoptosis* (cell death) in gastric cancer cell lines and decreased growth of liver cancer in rats. Two large cohort studies of over 130,000 Chinese men and women showed that high intakes of celery decreased the risk of liver cancer, a malignancy very common in China.

90

Bibliography

- Gao LL, Feng L, Yao ST, et al. Molecular mechanisms of celery seed extract induced *apoptosis* via S-phase cell cycle arrest in the BGC-823 human stomach cancer cell line. Asian Pac J Cancer Prev 2011;12:2601-2606

- Kuo CH, Weng BC, Yang SF, et al. Apigenin has anti-atrophic gastritis and anti-gastric cancer progression effects in *Helicobacter pylori*-infected Mongolian gerbils. J Ethnopharmacol 2014;151:1031-1039

- Sowbhagya HR. Chemistry, technology, and nutraceutical functions of celery (*Apium graveolens L.*): an overview. Crit Rev Food Sci Nutr 2014;54:389-398

- Sultana S, Ahmed S, Jahangir T, et al. Inhibitory effect of celery seeds extract on chemically induced hepatocarcinogenesis: modulation of cell proliferation, metabolism, and altered hepatic foci development. Cancer Lett 2005;221:11-20

- Zhang W, Xiang YB, Li HL, et al. Vegetable based dietary pattern and liver cancer risk: results from the Shanghai women's and mens' health studies. Cancer Sci 2013;104:1353-1361

- Zheng GQ, Kennedy PM, Zhang J, et al. Chemoprevention of benzo(a)pyrene-induced forestomach cancer in mice by natural phthalides from celery seed oil. Nutr Cancer 1993;19:77-86

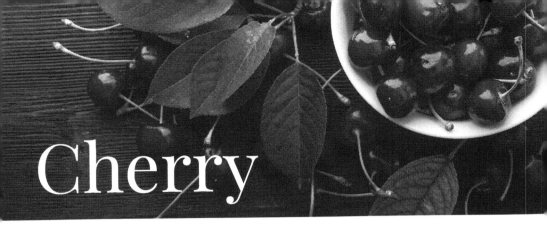

Cherry

Background

The cherry is a tree drupe, or "stone fruit", belonging to the genus *Prunus*. The sour or tart cherry (*P. cerasus*) and the sweet cherry (*P. avium*) are the most widely consumed varieties. The cherry is grown worldwide and can be eaten fresh, frozen, dried, or juiced. Cherries are often consumed as a dessert or added to fruit salads. Recently, research has identified potent anticancer properties present in cherries.

Anticancer properties

As cherries ripen from green to red, there is an accumulation of phytonutrients known as anthocyananins, which impart the characteristic color. Various antioxidant polyphenols are present in the skin and include cyanidins, pelagonidins, and hydroxycinnamates. Flavonols such as catechin, quercetin, and kaempferol are found in sweet and sour cherries, but total phenolic content is higher in the sour variety. Cherries possess significant antioxidant capacity when assessed with various laboratory assays. Proposed anticancer effects include increased plasma antioxidant capacity, increases in antioxidant enzyme activity in various tissues, and decreased systemic inflammation via decreasing tumor necrosis factor, cyclooxygenase, and nitric oxide — chemicals all produced in the body that can lead to inflammation resulting in cellular damage and cancer. Cell cultures of colon, liver, breast, and leukemia cells have shown that anthocyanins from cherries are anticarcinogenic. Additionally, anthocyanins induce cancer cell death (*apoptosis*) and block several pathways that cause cancer cells to proliferate (e.g., PI3K, ERK, and MAPK pathways).

Bibliography

- Damar I, Eski A. Antioxidant capacity and anthocyanin profile of sour cherry (*Prunus cerasus L.*) juice. Food Chem 2012;135:2910-2914

- Ferretti G, Baechetti T, Belleggia A, et al. Cherry antioxidants: from farm to table. Molecules 2010;15:6993-7005

- Martin KR, Wooden A. Tart cherry juice induces differential dose-dependant effects on *apoptosis*, but not cellular proliferation, in MCF-7 human breast cancer cells. J Med Food 2012;15:945-954

- McCune LM, Kubota C, Stendell-Hollis NR, et al. Cherries and health: a review. Crit Rev Food Sci Nutr 2011;51:1-12

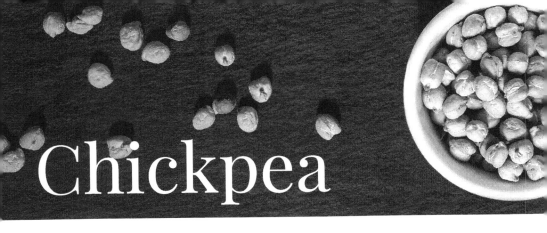

Chickpea

Background

Chickpea (*Cicer arietinum*), also known as a "pulse" crop, is grown and consumed worldwide. The chickpea has a long history, and is one of the ancient founder crops of the Fertile Crescent of the Near East. Grown in over fifty countries spanning all major continents, the chickpea forms a staple in many culture's diet, due to abundant amino acid profile, culinary versatility, and low cost. Recently, the chickpea has been noted to potentially decrease the risk of certain cancers.

Anticancer properties

The chickpea contains a variety of phytonutrients, antioxidants, and fatty acids that may improve overall health and inhibit neoplasia. Carotenoids (e.g., lycopene, beta-carotene, lutein) are lipid-soluble antioxidants that impart a yellow to red color in various plants, scavenge free-radicals and decrease cell damage. The isoflavone, biochanin A, found in chickpea, has been noted in animal studies to decrease epithelial tumor growth as well as to decrease lipid peroxidation, a process that leads to cell injury and cancer. Lycopene, a carotenoid that imparts a deep-red color to tomatoes and watermelon, is a potent antioxidant that also decreases cell damage and inhibits proliferation. When chickpeas (and other beans) reach the colon, butyrate, a short chain fatty acid (SCFA), is produced. Butyrate suppresses cell proliferation and inhibits DNA damage within the colonic cells. *Beta*-sistosterol, a fat-containing phytochemical found in chickpea, has been shown to inhibit colon carcinogenesis in rats fed N-methyl-N-nitrosurea.

94

Intake of carotenoids has been shown to reduce prostate cancer growth in animals. Additionally, carotenoid intake in general, has been associated with a decreased risk of lung and other epithelial cancers in humans. Biochanin A inhibited the growth of stomach cancer cells in mice and the SCFA butyrate is linked to a decreased risk of colon cancer.

Bibliography

- Bartley GE, Scolnik PA. Plant carotenoids: pigments for photoprotection, visual protection, and human health. Plant Cell 1995;7:1027-1038

- Bendich A. Recent advances in clinical research involving carotenoids. Pure Appl Chem 1994;66:1017-1024

- Jukanti AK, Gaur PM, Gowda CLL, et al. Nutritional quality and health benefits of chickpea (*Cicer arietinum*): a review. Br J Nutr 2012;108:S11-S26

- Raicht RF, Cohen BI, Fazzini EP, et al. Protective effect of plant sterols against chemically induced colon tumors in rats. Cancer Res 1980;40:403-405

- Yanaginara K, Ito A, Toge T, et al. Antiproliferative effects of isoflavones on human cancer cell lines established from the gastrointestinal tract. Cancer Res 1993;53:5815-5821

Chili Pepper

Background

The genus *Capsicum* refers to a group of plants that yield a variety of fruits commonly known as peppers. There are numerous varieties that range from large to small, mild to hot, and green to brilliant red. Two of the most widely used products of this genus include chili powder (dried and ground, often from hot peppers) and paprika (dried and ground large red peppers). The genus *Capsicum* contains an antioxidant compound known as capsaicin, which is responsible for the "heat" associated with a variety of peppers. Fruits of this genus are used worldwide in a variety of cuisines. In recent years, capsaicin has been studied for its effect on a variety of illnesses, including a potential role in cancer prevention.

Anticancer properties

Capsaicin has been demonstrated to impart an antiproliferative effect on various cancer cells *in vitro*. Capsaicin induced *apoptosis* (cell death) in human breast and leukemia cell lines in one study. Inhibition of various cancer-promoting pathways such as NF-kB, STAT3, and COX has been attributed to capsaicin. Capsaicin has been demonstrated to inhibit generation of benzo(a)pyrene, a carcinogen found in cigarette smoke. Some studies have shown capsaicin to inhibit proliferation and/or induce *apoptosis* of esophagus, stomach, lung, prostate, and liver cancer cells. Some authors have demonstrated that the combination of green tea extract and capsicum extract induces synergistic inhibition of different cancer cell lines

Bibliography

- Dou D, Ahmad A, Yang H, Sarkar FH. Tumor cell growth inhibition is correlated with levels of capsaicin present in hot peppers. Nutr Cancer 2011;63:272-281

- Dwivedi V, Shrivastava R, Hussain S, et al. Cytotoxic potential of Indian spices (extracts) against esophageal squamous carcinoma cells. Asian Pacific J Cancer Prev 2011;12:2069-2073

- Oyagbemi AA, Saba AB, Azeez OI. Capsaicin: a novel chemopreventative molecule and its underlying molecular mechanisms of action. Indian J Cancer 2010;47:53-58

Citrus Peel

Background

Citrus fruits are well-known for their health-promoting properties and contain a significant amount of the antioxidant vitamin, ascorbic acid (vitamin C). Deficiency of vitamin C results in scurvy, now uncommon in the Western world, a life-threatening disorder of collagen function that can lead to severe bleeding. Oranges, limes, and lemons contain significant amounts not only of vitamin C, but also anticancer phytonutrients. Sweet orange (*Citrus sinensis*) peel is available in dried form and may hold potential as an anticancer agent when added to the diet.

Anticancer properties

Orange peel contains a variety of phytonutrients of which include the polymethoxy-flavones, a group of antioxidant flavonoids. Polymethoxyflavones from orange peel have been shown to inhibit proliferation and induce *apoptosis* (cell death) of human breast and lung cancer cell lines. Other flavonoids in orange peels such as hesperidin, naringenin, and naringin can also induce *apoptosis* and decrease growth of various cancer cell lines. Orange and other citrus peels possess free radical scavenging ability which may prevent cell damage that leads to cancer. Orange peel extract decreased colon cancer cell growth in mice in one study. Limonene is a phytochemical present in orange and other citrus peels that seemed to lower the risk of squamous cell skin cancer in an Arizona population study.

Bibliography

- Fan K, Kurihara N, Abe S, et al. Chemopreventative effects of orange peel extract (OPE): OPE inhibits intestinal tumor growth in ApcMin/+ mice. J Med Food 2007;10:11-17

- Hakim IA, Harris RB, Ritenbaugh C. Citrus peel use is associated with reduced risk of squamous cell carcinoma of the skin. Nutr Cancer 2000;37:161-168

- Meiyanto E, Hermawan A, Anindyajiti. Natural products for cancer-targeted therapy: citrus flavonoids as potent chemopreventive agents. Asian Pac J Cancer Prev 2012;13:427-436

- Sergeev IN, Ho CT, Colby J, et al. *Apoptosis*-inducing activity of hydroxylated polymethoxyflavones and polymethoxyflavones from orange peel in human breast cancer cells. Mol Nutr Food Res 2007;51:1478-1484

- Xiao H, Yang CS, Li S, et al. Monodemethylated polymethoxyflavones from sweet orange (*Citrus sinensis*) peel inhibit growth of human lung cancer cells by *apoptosis*. Mol Nutr Food Res 2009;53:398-406

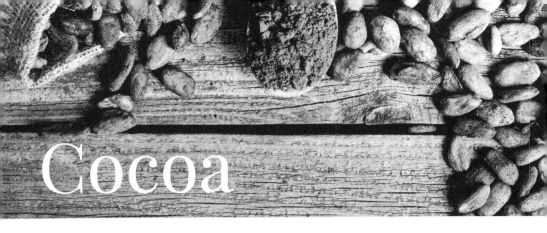

Cocoa

Background

Cocoa, the seed of the cocoa tree (*Theobroma cacao*), is best-known for being the central ingredient in the ever-popular indulgence food, chocolate. Cocoa has been enjoyed from at least 600 years B.C. and continues to be a heavily consumed food throughout the world in the form of solid chocolate, cocoa liquor, and cocoa powder. Recently, cocoa has been demonstrated to possess health-promoting anticancer compounds known as polyphenols, which are especially abundant in darker chocolates.

Anticancer properties

Cocoa contains antioxidant compounds known as polyphenols. Cell-damaging free radicals are produced *via* normal cellular metabolism and contain oxygen molecules that induce damage not only to the outer cell membrane, but also to DNA. Cancer may result with ongoing DNA damage from these free-radicals. Polyphenols constitute a large class of antioxidant compounds with cocoa being abundant in catechins, epicatechin, gallic acid, and procyanidins. Cocoa powder and dark chocolate contain the highest amounts of antioxidants compared to milk chocolate, which contains approximately one-half the amount of dark chocolate. Laboratory studies have shown that cocoa polyphenols inhibit the cell-damaging effects of the cell-poison, peroxynitrate and superoxide radical — chemicals formed by immune cells in response to normal ongoing cell damage within the body. Cocoa also contains 2-3% theobromine, which possesses antioxidant activity.

There are few data with regards to prevention of specific cancers by cocoa, but laboratory and epidemiologic studies suggest that polyphenol intake from fruits and vegetables can inhibit cancer cell growth in the laboratory, in animals, and possibly, humans. More research is necessary to ascertain how much cocoa may be necessary to prevent certain cancers. Nonetheless, cocoa is another way to increase the total antioxidant load in the diet.

Bibliography

- Cooper KA, Donovan JL, Waterhouse AL, et al. Cocoa and health: a decade of research. British J Nutr 2008;99:1-11

- Jalil AM, Ismail A. Polyphenols in cocoa and cocoa products: is there a link between antioxidant properties and health? Molecules 2008;13:2190-2219

- Lee KW, Kim YJ, Lee HJ, et al. Cocoa has more phenolic phytochemicals and a higher antioxidant capacity than teas and red wine. J Agric Food Chem 2003;51:7292-7295

- Ramiro-Puig E, Catell M. Cocoa: antioxidant and immunomodulator. Br JNutr 2009;101:931-940

- Weisburger JH. Chemopreventive effects of cocoa polyphenols on chronic diseases. Exper Biol Med 2001;226:891-897

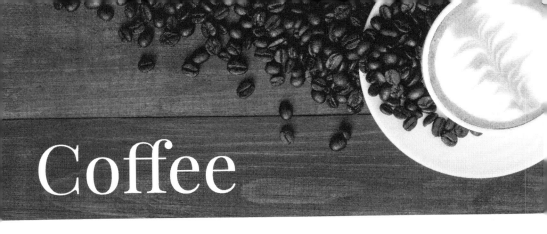

Coffee

Background

Next to tea, coffee is perhaps the most widely consumed beverage in the world. Coffee is cultivated throughout the world and despite negative press over the years with regards to possible cancer-causing properties, coffee has been increasingly recognized as being rich in numerous antioxidants which may prevent certain cancers and prevent chronic diseases such as diabetes.

Anticancer properties

Coffee contains numerous antioxidant compounds, notably flavanoids, phenols (e.g., chlorogenic acids and cinnamic acids), and diterpines (e.g., cafestol and kahweol), which have been demonstrated in laboratory and animal studies to decrease formation of cell-damaging oxidants and free-radicals such as superoxide, hydrogen peroxide, hydroxyl radical, peroxyl radical, and peroxynitrate. These endogenously-derived chemicals damage cell membranes and DNA, which can increase the risk of various cancers. Coffee has also been shown to reduce carcinogen formation and subsequent cell damage in animal studies. Kwon and colleagues utilized an elegant laboratory assay that demonstrated dose-dependent inhibition of peroxyl radical generation by various beverages, especially brewed and instant coffee. Both forms of coffee were active antioxidants with a cup of brewed coffee demonstrating peroxyl radical scavenging activity exceeding the capacity provided by the recommended daily dose of vitamin C. In fact, studies have shown that regular coffee intake influences plasma antioxidant capacity in human subjects. Additionally, the stimulant caffeine has been shown to directly suppress tumor formation in some studies, especially colon cancer cell growth.

Despite early reports of increased risk of pancreatic and bladder cancer linked to coffee, recent studies have *not* confirmed that coffee causes cancer. Experiments in laboratory animals have demonstrated a lower risk of colon and rectal cancers with coffee administration. Recent epidemiologic data in humans has shown variable decreased risk of cancers of the breast, colon, rectum, kidney, and liver in various populations. A Japanese study revealed an especially strong association between coffee intake and a reduced risk of liver cancer, with a risk reduction of 76% in persons who drank more than five cups daily compared to non-drinkers. Premenopausal women have up to a 20% reduced risk of breast cancer with regular coffee intake. Patients treated for stage III colon cancer have a lower risk of reoccurrence if they drink 4 or more cups daily.

Bibliography

- Cavin C, Holzhaeuser D, Scharf G, et al. Cafestol and kahweol, two coffee specific diterpenes with anticarcinogenic activity. Food Chem Toxicol 2002;40:1155-1163

- Guercio BJ, Sato K, Niedzwieckin, et al. Coffe intake, reoccurence, and mortality in stage III colon cancer: results from CALGB 89803. J Clin Oncol 2015;33:3598-3607

- Inoue M, Yoshimi I, Sobue T, et al. Influence of coffee drinking on subsequent risk of hepatocellular carcinoma: a prospective study in Japan. J Nat Cancer Inst 2005;97:293-300

- Jacobsen BK, Bjelke E, Kvale G, et al. Coffee drinking, mortality, and cancer incidence: results from a Norwegian prospective study. J Nat Cancer Inst 1986;76:823-831

- Kwon DY, Choi KH, Kim SJ, et al. Comparison of peroxyl radical scavenging capacity of commonly consumed beverages. Arch of Pharmacol Res 2009;32:283-287

- Natells F, Nardini M, Giannetti I, et al. Coffee drinking influences plasma antioxidant capacity in humans. J Agric Food Chem 2002;50:6211-6216

- Nkondjock A. Coffee consumption and the risk of cancer: an overview. Cancer Lett 2009;277:121-125

Coriander

Background

Coriander (*Corriandrum sativum*) is an ancient plant prized for its aromatic leaves and pungent seed pods. Coriander is mentioned in the Old Testament and is what "manna", a food that God fed the Israelites, was reported to resemble (Numbers 11:7). Coriander has been used medicinally for millennia and is indigenous to the Mediterranean region, but is also grown in Russia, Europe, Asia, and North Africa. Many cultures use coriander in their cuisine, and is an integral component of curry powder in India. Coriander is rich in phytochemicals and oils which may prevent cancer. As such, many studies have been conducted which have shown interesting results.

Anticancer properties

The fruit of coriander consists of a seed and pericarp which are rich in essential and fatty oils of which include various glycolipids, linoleic acid, palmitic acid, oleic acid, and linalool. However, the most abundant oil is petroselinic acid, which seems to possess anticancer properties. A variety of phenolic compounds exhibit antioxidant activity. Coriander extracts protected against lipid peroxidation in mice with colon cancer in one study. Diabetic rats fed coriander powder were noted to be protected from peroxidative damage; the seeds also demonstrated free radical scavaging ability against superoxides and hydroxyl radicals. Corriander extract also exhibited an ability to impair breast cancer metastasis and induce cell cycle arrest and cell death (*apoptosis*) *in vitro*. In addition, coriander is rich in tocols, such as *gamma*-tocoperol, which possess antioxidant properties.

Bibliography

- Chithra V, Leelamma S. *Corriander sativum*—effect on lipid metabolism in 1,2 dimethyl hydrazine induced colon cancer. J Ethnopharmacol 2000;71:457-463

- Deepa B, Anuradha CV. Antioxidant potential of *Coriandrum sativum* L. seed extract. Indian J Exp Biol 2011;49:30-38

- Sahib NG, Anwar F, Gilani AH, et al. Coriander (*Coriander sativum* L.): a potential source of high value components for functional foods and nutraceuticals—a review. Phytother Res 2013;10:1439-1456

- Tang EL, Rajarajeswaran J, Fung SY, et al. Antioxidant activity of *Coriander sativum* and protection against DNA damage and cancer cell migration. BMC Complement Altern Med 2013;13:347

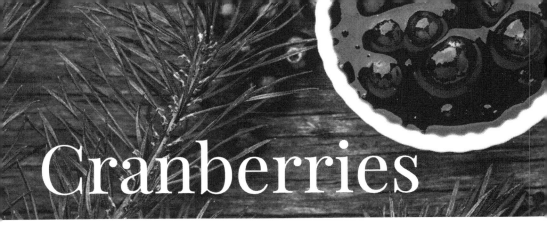

Cranberries

Background

The cranberry (*Vaccinium macrocarpon*), a close relative of the blueberry, is perhaps best known for the appearance it makes at Thanksgiving. However, increasing research suggests that this often "overlooked" food may prevent certain types of cancer as well as the ability of the juice to prevent urinary tract infections. Cranberries are water-loving plants that are grown in bogs and harvested as they float upon the water surface.

Anticancer properties

Like blueberries, cranberries contain numerous phytochemicals that have be shown experimentally to inhibit the growth of cancer cells. Proanthocyanidins and the similar anthocyanins which impart the fruit's color, have been demonstrated to decrease cancer cell growth, increase cancer cell death (*apoptosis*), inhibit tumor vessel growth (angiogenesis), inhibit the ability of cancer cells to detach from the tumor and spread (metastasize), and detoxify cancer causing compounds known as carcinogens. Inhibition of matrix metalloproteinases by cranberry extract diminishes the ability of cancer cells to erode out of the tumor into the bloodstream. Proanthocyanidins are more potent antioxidants than vitamins E or C, and slow or prevent growth of leukemia, oral, prostate, and lung cancer cells. Quecertin is also abundant in cranberries and possesses similar anticancer properties and inhibits *in vitro* growth of breast, colon, pancreas, and leukemia cells. Cranberry juice has been shown to impair lymphoma growth in mice. Other compounds in cranberries that may reduce tumor growth include triterpenoids, ellagitannins, phenolic acids, and stilbenoids. Although population-based studies are lacking, based on laboratory research, cranberries may decrease the risk of colorectal, breast, prostate, and lung cancers, as well as lymphoma. A recent human study revealed that cranberry juice decreased bacterial infection of the stomach with *Helicobacter pylori*, a bacteria responsible for causing stomach cancers. Excess or supplemental cranberry can cause kidney stones or interact with warfarin.

Bibliography

- Hochman N, Houri-Haddad Y, Koblinski J, et al. Cranberry juice constituents impair lymphoma growth and augment the generation of antilymphoma antibodies in syngenic mice. Nutr Cancer 2008;60:511-517

- Nandakumar V, Singh T, Katiyar SK. Multi-targeted prevention and therapy of cancer by proanthocyanidins. Cancer Lett 2008;269:378-387

- Neto CC. Cranberry and its phytochemicals: a review of *in vitro* anticancer studies. J Nutr 2007;137:186S-193S

- Neto CC. Cranberry and blueberry: evidence for protective effects against cancer and vascular diseases. Molec Nutr Food Res 2007;51:652-664

- Yan X, Murphy BT, Hammond GB, et al. Antioxidant activities and antitumor screening of extracts from cranberry fruit (*Vaccinium macrocarpon*). J Agric Food Chem 2002;50:5844-5849

Cumin Seed

Background

Cumin (*Cuminum cyminum*) is one of the earliest grown spices in Asia, Europe, and Africa. The seeds have been used in folklore and medicine for hundreds of years in many countries. Cumin seeds possess a very pungent aromatic property that lends well to many cuisines, notably in India. Cumin is mentioned in the Bible (Isaiah 28:27). This seed enjoys a prominent place in some cultures, in which cumin seed is kept in its own container on the table, similar to pepper.

Anticancer properties

Cumin contains numerous phytonutrients and essential oils. Cuminaldehyde is responsible in large part for the distinctive aroma and is a potent antioxidant. Other compounds present in cumin include linalool, pyrazines, terpinene, pinene, cymene, and safranal. Many authors have studied the phytonutrients in cumin and have noted anticancer properties. Cumin possesses antioxidant properties that can protect against cellular damage and quench free radicals formed during normal cellular metabolism. Cumin has been shown to decrease colon, cervix, stomach, and liver cancer growth in rodents. It has also been demonstrated to up-regulate production of the detoxifying enzyme, glutathione S-transferase and increase levels of the antioxidant enzymes, superoxide dismutase and catalase. Other laboratory experiments have shown that cumin antioxidants can scavenge hydroxyl- and peroxy- free radicals. The lower incidence of some cancers in India may be attributable to cumin ingestion.

Bibliography

- Aruna K, Sivaramakrishnan VM. Anticarcinogenic effects of some Indian plant products. Food Chem Toxicol 1992;30:953-956

- Gagandeep, Dhanalaksshmi S, Mendiz E, et al. Chemopreventative effects of *Cuminum cyminum* in chemically induced forestomach and uterine cervix tumors in murine model systems. Nutr Cancer 2003;47:171-180

- Johri RK. *Cuminum cyminum* and *carum carvi*: an update. Pharamcogn Rev 2011;5:63-72

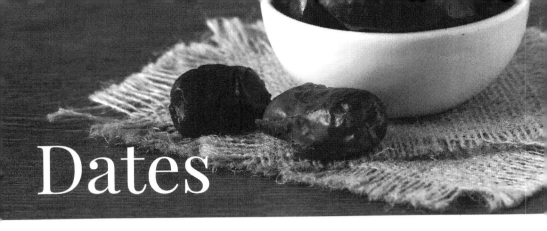

Dates

Background

  The date palm fruit (*Phoenix dactylifera*) is an ancient fruit that comes from one of the oldest trees grown and raised by humans. The date is believed by some to have originated in Mesopotamia (which includes modern-day Iraq) as early as 4000 B.C. Dates were consumed in Old Testament times and are mentioned in the Bible (2 Samuel 6:19, I Chronicles 16:3). During the Islamic Holiday of Ramadan, dates are eaten nightly to break the end of the long daily fasts. Date fruits have been purported to possess many medical and health-promoting properties and used as a dietary staple in the Middle East for thousands of years. The date palm is a member of the palm tree family, which grows in warm climates. Dates are a major crop of various countries such as Egypt and Saudi Arabia, but also grow in warmer regions of the United States.

Anticancer properties

  Dates have been believed to possess many health-enhancing properties including analgesic, antibacterial, anti-inflammatory, antidiabetic, and anticancer effects. Dates also contain vitamins, minerals, fiber, and have a low glycemic index despite being very sweet. Dates have been shown by researchers to contain several types of phytonutrients such as procyanidins, alkaloids, flavanoids, phenols, terpenoids, and tannins. Quercetin and apiginin are flavanoids that have been shown to decrease cancer cell growth in laboratory studies. The phenolic compounds have been shown to act as antioxidants, acting as scavengers of cell-damaging free radicals. A compound known as *beta* D-glucan found in date fruit suppressed tumor growth in laboratory studies.

Bibliography

- Al-Shabib W, Marshall RJ. The fruit of the date palm: its possible use for the best food for the future. Int J Food Sci Nutr 2003;54:247-259

- Ishurd O, Zgheel F, Kermagi A, et al. Antitumor activity of *beta*-D-glucan from Libyan dates. J Med Food 20047:252-255

- Rahmani AH, Aly SM, Ali H, et al. Therapeutic effects of date fruits (*Phoenix dactylifera*) in the prevention of diseases via modulation of anti-inflammatory, anti-oxidant and anti-tumor activity. Int J Clin Exp Med 2014;7:483-491

- Vayali PK. Date fruits (*Phoenix dactylifera Linn*): an emerging medicinal food. Crit Rev Food Sci Nutr 2012;52:249-271

Fennel Seed

Background

Fennel (*Foeniculum vulgare*) is a plant indigenous to the shores of the Mediterranean Sea but also grows along coastlines and rivers. Fennel is often used for the root bulb or leaves, but the seeds are a versatile ingredient especially utilized in India, Pakistan, and the Middle East. Fennel seed exudes a licorice-like taste and odor similar to anise, both of which contain anethole. Fennel seed is commonly ground and added to many dishes but also is used medicinally, often as a carminative (anti-gas agent) or a mild laxative. Recently, phytochemicals in fennel have been found to possess anticancer properties.

Anticancer properties

Fennel seed contains many phytochemicals including flavonoids, terpenoids, phenols, sterols, and alkaloids. Anethole is the key component of fennel seed that has been shown to inhibit inflammation and cancer growth as well as increase levels of the intracellular antioxidant, glutathione. Fennel extracts containing anethole inhibited the growth of adenocarcinoma cells in laboratory studies by blocking various enzymes and proteins involved in cancer cell proliferation. Fennel extract also inhibited growth of breast cancer and liver cancer cell lines *in vitro* and demonstrates the ability to scavenge free radicals.

Bibliography

- Aggarwal BB, Kunnumakkara AB, Harikumar KB, et al. Potential of spice-derived phytochemicals for cancer prevention. Planta Med 2008;74:1560-1569

- Mohamad RH, El-Bastawesy AM, Abel-Monem MG, et al. Antioxidant and anticarcinogenic effects of methanolic extract and volatile oil of fennel seeds (*Foeniculum vulgare*). J Med Food 2011;986-1001

- Skrovankova S, Misurcova L, Machu L. Antioxidant activity and protecting health effects of common medicinal plants. Adv Food Nutr Res 2012;67:75-139

Flaxseed

Background

    Flaxseed (*Linum usitatissimum*) is the edible seed of the ancient flax plant, and is a rich source of dietary fiber, beneficial fatty acids, and anticancer phytochemicals. Flaxseeds are also known as "oilseeds" due to their high content of various oil compounds, especially α-linolenic acid, an *omega-3* fatty acid similar to heart-healthy fatty acids found in cold-water fish. Recently, flaxseed has been shown to possess some interesting anticancer properties, especially against breast cancer—the most common malignancy amongst American women.

Anticancer properties

    Flaxseed contains high amounts of *omega-3* α-linolenic acid and lignans, a large family of fiber-related phenolic, antioxidant compounds that are found in a variety of plants. Linolenic acid is converted into secoisolariciresonol diglycoside (SDG), the dominant precursor to the human lignans, enterolactone and enterodiol, which have been shown experimentally to decrease the formation and growth of breast cancer cells. These lignans have been shown in laboratory animals to decrease the synthesis and release of various cancer growth-promoting compounds such as epidermal growth factor, insulin-like growth factor, and vascular endothelial growth factor. Lignans also block the effect of circulating estrogen, a hormone that stimulates breast cancer cell growth. Experiments in mice fed diets rich flaxseed have shown a decrease in the growth and spread of surgically-implanted breast cancer and melanoma tissue. Mice fed flaxseed also have decreased formation and growth of prostate as well as precancerous colon cancer cells. Lignans may also inhibit the growth of blood vessels into tumors, thereby depriving the cancer of blood and oxygen. Flaxseed supplementation has been shown to decrease the risk of breast, colon, prostate, and melanoma cancers in rodents. Demark-Wahnefried and colleagues administered a flaxseed-supplemented diet (30 grams daily) to patients with prostate cancer for 30 days prior to surgery and found evidence of decreased cancer cell growth in the operative specimens. This provides proof-of-principle that daily consumption of flaxseed may reduce the growth of human cancer.

Bibliography

- Bergman JM, Thomson LU, Dabrosin C. Flaxseed and its lignans inhibit estradiol-induced growth, angiogenesis, and secretion of vascular endothelial growth factor in human breast cancer xenografts *in vivo*. Clin Cancer Res 2007;13:1061-1067

- Chen J, Wang L, Thompson LU. Flaxseed and its components reduce metastasis after surgical excision of solid human breast tumor in nude mice. Cancer Lett 2006;234:168-175

- Denmark-Wahnefried W, Polascik TJ, George SL, et al. Flaxseed supplementation (not dietary fat restriction) reduces prostate cancer proliferation rates in men presurgery. Cancer Epidemiol Biomark Prev 2008;17:3577-3587

- Saarinen NM, Warri A, Airio M, et al. Role of dietary lignans in the reduction of breast cancer risk. Mol Nutr Food Res 2007;51:857-866

- Williams D, Verghese M, Walker LT, et al. Flax seed oil and flax seed meal reduce the formation of aberrant crypt foci (ACF) in azoxymethane-induced colon cancer in Fisher 344 male rats. Food Chem Toxicol 2007;45:153-159

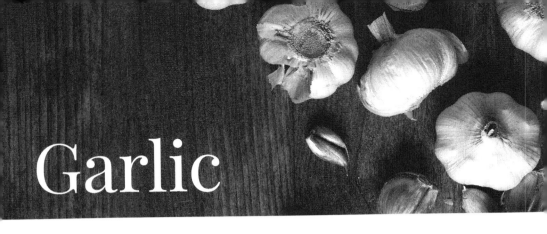

Garlic

Background

Garlic, *Allium sativum*, is known for a pungent smell that adds unique flavor to a variety of foods. In the same family as onions, leeks, and chives, garlic grows in head-like clusters containing individual pods surrounded by a durable, fibrous peel. When crushed or cut, a compound known as allicin is released and gives rise to the peculiar odor of garlic. Ancient societies of China, Egypt, and Greece utilized garlic for perceived medicinal properties. However, recent epidemiologic studies have suggested that garlic may possess cancer-fighting properties.

Anticancer properties

The pungent odor and anticancer properties of garlic result from sulfur-containing chemicals such as diallyl sulfide, disulfides, trisulfides, allyl mercaptan, and allyl methyl sulfide. These, and may other compounds may inhibit cancer cell growth by a variety of mechanisms such as induction of cell death (*apoptosis*), disrupted cancer cell metabolism, decreased cell growth and proliferation, decreased tumor vessel growth (angiogenesis), and scavenging of free radicals—oxygen-containing chemicals that damage DNA. Carcinogens are chemicals that are acquired through the environment (through inhalation or ingestion) that often require activation within cells into cancer-causing compounds. Numerous carcinogens causing a variety of cancers in a laboratory rodents have been inhibited by garlic extracts. Garlic has also been shown to experimentally prevent DNA damage as well as aid in DNA repair. Allyl compounds decrease tumor proliferation in experimental models of lymphoma, skin, esophagus, breast, prostate, and lung cancer. Garlic may also enhance function of immune cells such as lymphocytes, natural killer cells, and macrophages, which destroy cancer cells.

Population-based studies provide evidence that certain human malignancies may be prevented by regular garlic ingestion. A study of 42,000 women in Iowa aged 55-69 demonstrated that garlic consumption was associated with a decreased risk of cancer overall and, in particular, a 50% lower risk of colon cancer compared to women who did not consume garlic. Studies in Northern China where garlic production is high, reveal a decreased incidence of stomach cancer compared to the rest of the country. Limited evidence for prevention of colon, prostate, esophageal, throat, mouth, ovary, and kidney cancers has been shown in several studies.

Bibliography

- Craig WJ. Health-promoting properties of common herbs. American Journal of Clinical Nutrition 1999;70:491S-499S

- Khanum F, Anilakumar KR, Viswanathan KR. Anticarcinogenic properties of garlic: a review. Crit Rev Food Sci Nutr 2004;44:479-488

- Milner JA. Preclinical perspectives on garlic and cancer. J Nutr 2006;136:827S-831S

- Milner JA. Garlic: its anticarcinogenic and antitumorigenic properties. Nutr Rev 1996;54:82-86

- Milner JA. A historical perspective on garlic and cancer. J Nutr 2001;131:1027S-1031S

- Pinto JT, Rivlin RS. Antiproliferative effects of *allium* derivatives of garlic. J Nutr 2001;131:1058S-1060S

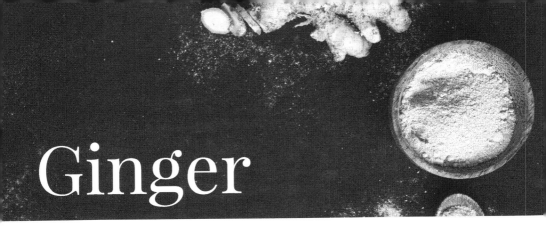

Ginger

Background

Ginger is the rhizome, or tuberous root, of *Zingiber officianalis*, is a fascinating plant with significant history. Ginger has been consumed and utilized for medicinal purposes for centuries and is now receiving much attention due to a myriad of health-promoting properties. Ginger has been used for over 2500 years in China and is still commonly used as a functional herb or medicine for innumerable health conditions in various Asian cultures. Interestingly, population-based studies have demonstrated a decreased incidence of a variety of cancers compared to the United States, which has been attributed, at least in part, to diets high in various phytonutrient-rich vegetables, fruits, legumes, and nuts. Ginger possesses several biologically active substances that have been shown to decrease cancer risk.

Anticancer properties

Ginger is complex biochemically, containing numerous phytonutrients including volatile and non-volatile compounds. Volatile oils include zingeberene, curcumene, and farnesene, and bisabolene; over 50 other volatile hydrocarbons have been isolated in smaller amounts and contribute to the characteristic pungent odor and taste. Non-volatile compounds predominant in ginger include gingerols, shogaols, paradols, and gingerone; these contribute to the pungency and "hot" characteristic of ginger. Gingerol is the most abundant antioxidant in ginger, and perhaps the most active. Numerous laboratory and animal studies have demonstrated that ginger and/or ginger extracts possess antioxidant and antiproliferative properties that decrease cancer cell formation and growth. Ginger can scavenge free radicals such as superoxide anions and induce *apoptosis* (cell death) of cancer cells as well as block various cancer cell proliferation pathways. Ginger has also been demonstrated to inhibit synthesis of inflammatory leukotrienes and prostaglandins, which increase the inflammatory mileau and can contribute to malignant cell transformation. Ginger extracts have been found to inhibit growth of lymphoma, leukemia, melanoma, colon, and breast cancer cells. Epidemiology studies suggest that countries with higher ginger intake may have a lower risk of a variety of cancers.

Bibliography

- Baliga MS, Haniadka R, Pereira MM, et al. Update on chemopreventive effects of ginger and its phytochemicals. Crit Rev Food Sci Nutr 2011;51:499-523

- Kundu JK, Na HK, Surh YJ. Ginger-derived phenolic substances with cancer preventive and therapeutic potential. Forum Nutr 2009;61:182-192

- Shukla Y, Singh M. Cancer preventative properties of ginger: a brief review. Food Chem Toxicol 2007;45:683-690

- Surh YJ, Lee E, Lee JM. Chemoprotective properties of some pungent ingredients present in red pepper and ginger. Mutation Research 1998;402:259-267

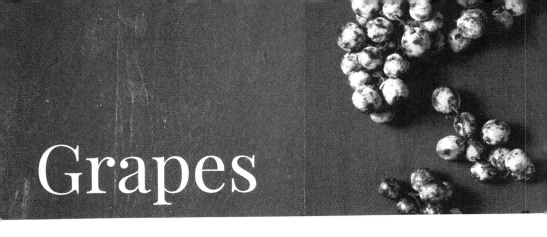

Grapes

Background

Grapevine (*Vitis vinifera*) products such as whole grapes, grape juice, wine, and raisins (dried grapes) are grown worldwide and play an integral part of the diet in many cultures. For instance, the Mediterranean diet, a diet rich in fruits, vegetables, olive oil, and red wine has been associated with a lower incidence of cardiac disease and certain cancers, which may in-part be due to constituents in grape products.

Anticancer properties

Grapes, especially dark skinned varieties, are a rich source of polyphenols — complex chemical structures that act as antioxidants and scavenge toxic free radicals. Inhibition of free-radical damage to cell membranes and DNA may prevent or slow the growth of various cancers. Free radicals are oxygen-containing compounds that are formed via normal cell reactions or by metabolism of environmental or ingested toxic substances. Grapes contain numerous polyphenols, with quercetin and resveratrol being the most abundant. Resveratrol is found in higher amounts in the skin of red or purple grapes; red wine, purple grape juice, and dark raisins also contain significant amounts. Resveratrol has been shown to decrease cancer cell growth and cause cell death (*apoptosis*) of skin, breast, colon, lung, esophagus, pancreas, prostate, and leukemia cells *in vitro* and in laboratory rodents. Since grape skin contains numerous other polyphenols, ingestion of the skin may be especially important since extracts of grape skin have shown more potent anticancer effects in laboratory studies.

Grapes in the form of juice, raisins, whole grapes, and red wine may decrease the risk of cancer overall, as demonstrated in many studies on the Mediterranean diet, in which consumption of not only red wine, but also raisins and grapes is commonplace. Some human studies have noted a lower risk of lung cancer in regular consumers of red wine, which may be an effect of resveratrol. If this is the case, consumption of other grape products such as juice, whole grapes, and raisins, could also lower the risk of lung cancer, although definitive evidence is lacking. A study in Korea demonstrated that consumption of a glass of grape juice daily for eight weeks by healthy volunteers resulted in higher blood levels of antioxidant activity and decreased DNA damage to circulating white blood cells. This study provides evidence that regular intake of grape products may decrease the risk of cancer in general.

Bibliography

- Athar M, Back JH, Tang X, et al. Resveratrol: a review of pre-clinical studies for human cancer prevention. Toxicol App Pharmacol 2007;224:274-283

- Castillo-Pichardo L, Martinez-Montemayor MM, Martinez JE, et al. Inhibition of mammary tumor growth and metastases to bone and liver by dietary grape polyphenols. Clin Exp Metastasis 2009;26:505-516

- Kaliora AC, Kountouri AM, Karathonos VT, et al. Effect of Greek raisins (*Vitis vinifera L*) from different origins on gastric cancer cell growth. Nutr Cancer 2008;60:792-799

- Morre DM, Morre DJ. Anticancer activity of grape and grape skin extracts alone and combined with green tea infusions. Cancer Lett 2006;238:202-209

- Park YK, Park E, Kim JS, et al. Daily grape juice consumption reduces oxidative DNA damage and plasma free radical levels in healthy Koreans. Mutational Res 2003;529:77-86

- Singletary KW, Stansbury MJ, Giusti M, et al. Inhibition of rat mammary tumorigenesis by concord grape juice constituents. J Agric Food Chem 2003;51:7280-7286

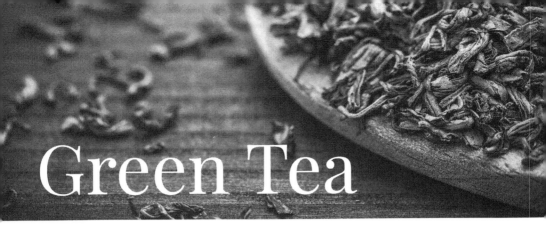

Green Tea

Background

Tea leaf is harvested from the *Camellia sinensis* bush and, next to water, is the most widely consumed beverage in the world. The major types of tea include black, green, and oolong, and are so-named depending on the preparation of the leaf. Green tea is immediately steamed after harvesting and not oxidized, so retains its pale green color and possesses several anticancer compounds. Green tea is the best studied of all tea varieties with regards to cancer-prevention.

Anticancer properties

Green tea contains approximately 40% dry weight of polyphenol compounds known as catechins. The major catechins found in green tea include epigallocatechin gallate (EGCG), epigallocatechin (ECG), and epicatechin which are the constituents that play a major role in the antioxidant and cancer-prevention effects. The average cup of green tea steeped for three minutes contains approximately 250-350 milligrams of tea solids, of which 30-40% are catechins. Epigallocatechin gallate is the most abundant and powerful antioxidant within green tea and possesses antioxidant activity 25-100 times more potent than vitamins C and E. Additionally, EGCG inhibits formation of metastasis and blood vessels in laboratory cancers and slows the growth of cancers in laboratory animals. Green tea has also been shown to decrease the rate of cancer cell proliferation and increase the rate of cell death (*apoptosis*) in human leukemia, breast, and prostate cancer cells *in vitro*. Green tea extract also possesses anticarcinogenic effects by inhibiting the formation of endogenous carcinogens and by breaking down those already formed. This may help to protect against DNA damage, which is a frequent event leading to cancer. Tests in human subjects have shown increased blood antioxidant activity in healthy people shortly after consuming 450 milliliters of green tea and decreased formation of plasma oxidants after daily consumption of one liter of green tea for four weeks. Interestingly, coadministration of green tea and capsicum (an antioxidant found in peppers) to *in vitro* cancer cells increased antioxidant activity synergistically compared to green tea extract alone.

Several epidemiologic studies have shown an inverse association between increased green tea intake and a decreased overall risk of cancer in several populations. Studies in Asia have shown that green tea may protect against the development of stomach cancer, the leading cause of cancer death in Japan. Increased green tea consumption has also been correlated with a decreased incidence of breast and lung cancers in some studies.

Bibliography

- Arts ICW. A review of the epidemiological evidence on tea, flavanoids, and lung cancer. J Nutr 2008;138:1561S-1566S

- Butt MS, Sultan MT. Green Tea: nature's defense against malignancies. Crit Rev Food Sci Nutr 2009;49:463-473

- Chen D, Dou QP. Tea polyphenols and their roles in cancer prevention and chemotherapy. Int J Mol Sci 2008;9:1196-1206

- Craig WJ. Health-promoting properties of common herbs. Am J Clin Nutr 1999;70:491S-499S

- Forney GB, Morre DJ, Morre DM. Oxidative stress reduced by green tea concentrate and *Capsicum* combination: synergistic effects. J Diet Suppl 2013;10:318-324

- Khan N, Mukhtar H. Multitargeted therapy of cancer by green tea polyphenols. Cancer Lett 2008;269:269-280

- Le Marchand L. Cancer preventive effects of flavonoids—a review. Biomed Pharmacother 2002;56:296-301

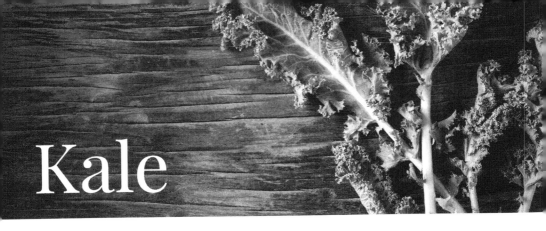

Kale

Background

    Brassica, or cuciferous, vegetables are closely-related vegetables all belonging to the genus and species, *Brassica oleracea*. Kale, is deep-green with thick leaves; broccoli and cauliflower both have a tumor-like appearance (hence the term, *botrytis,* which refers to a lobulated mass). Although these vegetables look quite different, their content of various phytochemicals and anticancer compounds are very similar. One similarity these vegetables possess is a pungent odor during cutting and cooking, which is attributed to the high sulfur content in the *Brassica* family.

Anticancer properties

    Brassica are abundant in a family of compounds known as isothiocyanates — sulfur-containing chemicals that are able to stop the conversion of carcinogens into DNA-damaging metabolites. Additionally, isothiocyanates convert dangerous chemicals, whether ingested toxins (e.g., cigarette smoke and radiation) or those generated within the body (e.g., electrophiles and reactive oxygen species), into compounds that are safely eliminated. Metastasis, spread of cancer, was inhibited by broccoli extract in laboratory breast cancer cells and is felt to be due to isothiocyanate activity. Cabbage fed to rats decreased the risk of chemically-induced breast tumors.

    Sulforaphane is one of many isothiocyanates (over 100) found in the *Brassica* family which has been shown in experiments to inhibit cancer cell growth. In laboratory experiments, sulforaphane has delayed cancer cell growth, stopped the conversion of various chemicals into carcinogens, and detoxified active carcinogens into safe metabolites for elimination. Furthermore, sulforaphane has slowed the growth or proliferation and caused death of cancer cells in laboratory studies. Using complex laboratory methods, Riso and colleagues demonstrated that a 200 gram serving of broccoli daily for ten days fed to 20 young healthy men (10 smokers) significantly reduced DNA damage in circulating blood cells in the smoking group.

The *Brassica* vegetables were associated with an observed 51% decrease in the development of bladder cancer in 47,909 men in the Health Professionals Follow-up Study published in 2001. Other population-based studies have demonstrated a reduction in the risk of prostate cancer, breast cancer, and lymphoma in women. *Brassicas* in general may decrease the risk of stomach colon, ovary, and uterus cancer.

Bibliography

- Beecher CWW. Cancer preventive properties of varieties of *Brassica oleracea*: a review. Am J Clin Nutr 1994;59:11665-11705

- Clarke JD, Dashwood RH, Ho E. Multi-targeted prevention of cancer by sulforaphane. Cancer Lett 2008;269:291-304

- Fahey JW, Zhang Y, Talalay P. Broccoli sprouts: an exceptionally rich source of inducers of enzymes that protect against chemical carcinogens. Proc Nat Acad Sci 1997;94:10367-10372

- Munday R, Mhawech-Fauceglia P, Munday CM, et al. Inhibition of urinary bladder carcinogenesis by broccoli sprouts. Cancer Res 2008;68:1593-1600

- Riso P, Martini D, Visioli F, et al. Effect of broccoli intake on markers related to oxidative stress and cancer risk in healthy smokers and nonsmokers. Nutr Cancer 2009;61:232-237

- Talalay P, Fahey JW. Phytochemicals from cruciferous plants protect against cancer by modulating carcinogen metabolism. J Nutr 2001;131:30275-30335

- Verhoeven DT, Goldbohm RA, van Poppel G, et al. Epidemiological studies on *brassica* vegetables and cancer risk. Cancer Epidemiol Biomark Prev 1996;5:733-748

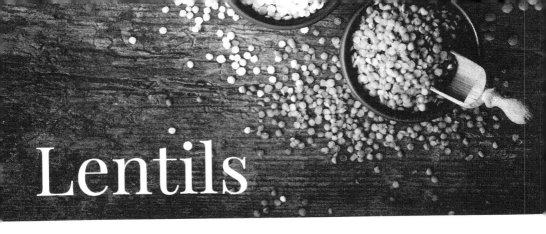

Lentils

Background

Lentils (*Lens culinaris*) are small disc-shaped legumes also known as a "pulse." Lentils have ancient roots, having been consumed for thousands of years, and exist in various colors, most commonly green, yellow, red, and black. They are staples of the Mediterranean region but also consumed in Asia and the Americas. Lentils are dense in protein and fiber, as well as easy to cook, making them a versatile ingredient in many cuisines. As such, they are a valuable addition to any diet, providing several phytonutrients.

Anticancer properties

Lentils are rich in phenolic compounds — potent antioxidants that prevent cell damage by scavenging free radicals and inhibiting damage to macromolecules within cells (e.g., lipids, proteins, and DNA). Amarowicz identified several phenolics within lentil extract such as quercetin, catechin, procyanindins, and hydroxybenzoic acid. Other experimental data have shown that lentil extracts possess significant antioxidant capacity. The fiber in lentil may also help decrease risk of colon cancer by increasing stool bulk and decreasing transit time, thereby limiting contact of bile acid-rich, carcinogenic feces with bowel tissue. A population-based cohort study in Japan showed that regular intake of legumes/lentils resulted in a 7-8% reduction in death among the age group of 70 years and above.

Bibliography

- Amarowicz R, Estrella I, Hernandez T, et al. Antioxidant activity of a red lentil extract and its fractions. Int J Mol Sci 2009;10:5513-5527

- Darmadi-Blackberry I, Wahlqvist ML, Kouris-Blazos A, et al. Legumes: the most important dietary predictor of survival in older people of different ethnicities. Asia Pac J Clin Nutr 2004;13:217-220

- Marathe SA, Rajalakshmi V, Jamdar SN, et al. Comparative study on antioxidant activity of different variety of commonly consumed legumes in India. Food Chem Toxicol 2011;49:2005-2012

- Zou Y, Chang SK, Gu Y, et al. Antioxidant activity and phenolic compositions of lentil (*Lens culinaris* var. Morton) extract and its fractions. J Agric Food Chem 2011;59:2268-2276

Maple Syrup

Background

Maple syrup is a thick, sugar-rich liquid that is extracted from the genus of maple (*Acer spp.*) trees. The maple tree is indigenous to North America and consists of numerous species. The sap of the maple tree has the consistency of water and is rich in sugars. The sap is heated and, eventually, a thicker material ensues—known as maple syrup. Maple syrup is widely used as a condiment for breakfast, but is also a flavorful and healthy alternative to table sugar as a general sweetener. Recent research has shown that maple syrup may be useful for cancer prevention.

Anticancer properties

Maple sap and syrup are rich in phytonutrients known as phenolics, which possess antiproliferative properties against a variety of cancer cells *in vitro*. For instance, maple sap/syrup extract contains phenolics known as ginnalins and maplexins that have been shown to stop DNA replication (known as the S-phase of cell division) in colon cancer cells. Maple syrup phenolics also inhibit colon and breast cancer cell growth by decreasing cyclin D1, a protein important in cancer cell proliferation. Maple syrup extract is also a fairly active antioxidant, and may protect cells from damage that can lead to cancerous transformation. Phillips and colleagues assessed antioxidant activities of sugar and alternative natural sweeteners and found that maple syrup has moderate antioxidant properties while refined sugar and corn syrup possessed nil antioxidant activity.

Bibliography

- Gonzalez GS, Li Liya, Seeram NP. Effects of Maple (*Acer*) plant part extracts on proliferation, *apoptosis*, and cell cycle arrest of human tumorigenic and non-tumorigenic colon cells. Phytother Res 2012;26:995-1002

- Gonzalez GS, Ma H, Edmonds ME, et al. Maple polyphenols, ginnalins A-C, induce S-and G2/M-cell cycle arrest in colon and breast cancer cells mediated by decreasing cyclins A and D1 levels. Food Chem 2013;136:636-642

- Gonzalez SA, Yuan T, Seeram NP. Cytoxicity and structure activity relationship studies of maplexins A-I, gallotannins from red maple (*Acer rubrum*). Food Chem Toxicol 2012;50:1369-1376

- Phillips KM, Carlsen MH, Blomhoff R. Total antioxidant content of alternatives to refined sugar. J Am Diet Assoc 2009;109:64-71

Mustard Seed

Background

Mustard (*Brassica species*) seeds are very small seeds from various types of mustard plants. Mustard seed is used in the cuisines of many cultures and has ancient tradition. In the New Testament, Jesus spoke of the mustard seed many times, comparing it to the Kingdom of Heaven (Matthew 13:31) and faith (Luke 17:6). Mustard seeds are used in the Middle and Far East in various dishes and in pickling. Additionally, the oil can be extracted and used for a variety of culinary indications. Recently, researchers have noted that mustard seed may inhibit the growth of cancer. Mustard seed has also gained attention because it is consumed in high amounts in Japan—the country with the longest life-expectancy in the world.

Anticancer properties

Mustard seed extracts have been found to prevent the growth of and induce *apoptosis* (cell death) of human colon cancer cells *in vitro*. Yuan and colleagues showed that mice fed diets enriched with mustard seeds lowered blood levels of malonaldehyde, a toxic by-product of cell damage, when the animals were fed carcinogens. This study also showed increased activity of various antioxidant systems (such as glutathione and superoxide dismutase) within the mice in a dose-dependent manner and decreased the risk of precancerous colon tumors. Other animal studies have demonstrated that mustard seed decreased the growth of bladder cancer and malignant colon tumors.

Bibliography

- Bhattacharya A, Li Y, Wade KL, et al. Allyl isothiocyanate-rich mustard seed powder inhibits bladder cancer growth and muscle invasion. Carcinogenesis. 2010;31:2105-2110

- Hashim S, Banerjee S, Mabhubala R, et al. Chemoprevention of DMBA-induced transplacental and translactational carcinogenesis in mice by oil from mustard seeds (*Brassica* spp.). Cancer Lett 1998;134:217-226

- Yuan H, Zhu M, Guo W, et al. Mustard seeds (*Sinappis alba Linn*) attenuate azoxymethane-induced colon carcinogenesis. Redox Rep 2011;16:38-44

- Zhu M, Yuan H, Guo W, et al. Dietary mustard seeds (*Sinapis alba Linn*) suppress 1,2-dimethylhydrazine-induced immune-imbalance and colonic carcinogenesis in rats. Nutr Cancer 2012;64:464-472

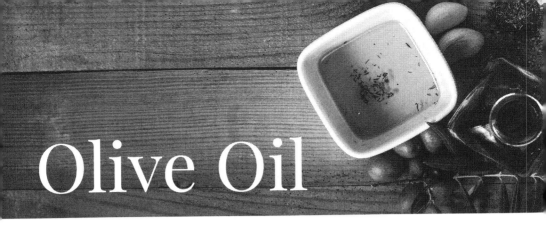

Olive Oil

Background

    The olive tree, *Olea europea*, requires stringent climatic conditions, with the majority of the world's olive supply coming from European countries bordering the Mediterranean Sea, such as Italy, Greece, and Spain. The olive is actually a drupe, a fruit consisting of a central seed (endocarp) surrounded by the pulp (mesocarp), and covered by skin (epicarp). Olive oil is expressed from the fruit by crushing whole olives in a hammer mill which results in a paste known as pomace that is pressed under high pressure between hydraulic plates. The expressed oil is filtered through a filter membrane. The oil, separated from the pomace and water, is centrifuged, leaving a product known as extra-virgin olive oil (EVOO), the highest quality of oil containing the most disease-modifying compounds. If this oil is again processed, lower quality virgin oil results. The so-called Mediterranean diet, consumed in much of Europe and associated with lower risks of heart disease and cancer, consists heavily of EVOO.

Anticancer properties

    Olive oil contains hundreds of disease-fighting compounds such as monounsaturated fatty acids, vitamin E, carotenes, and antioxidant phenol compounds. Oleic acid is the primary fatty acid found in olive oil and decreases cellular oxidative stress that can result in cancer. Vitamin E, *alpha*-tocopherol, acts as an antioxidant, as do compounds known as triterpenes. Phenol compounds in EVOO that may prevent cancer include secoiridoids, tyrosol, hydroxytyrosol, terpenoids, and lignans. Most of these antioxidant phenols are able to scavenge free radicals such as hydroxyl radical (·OH) and hydrogen peroxide (H_2O_2). Lignans, in particular, have been shown in experimental studies to slow growth of skin, colon, lung, and breast cancers. An interesting agent found in EVOO, known as squalene, is deposited in the skin, and may prevent skin cancers such as melanoma, by scavenging free radicals within the skin; rodent studies support this concept since squalene inhibits experimental skin cancers. Many of these antioxidants have been shown to scavenge free radicals in stool, which may protect against the formation of colon cancer. Secoiridoids and lignans were found to decrease growth of breast cancer cells in laboratory studies.

Population studies conducted in European countries that produce and consume large amounts of olive oil (e.g., Spain, Italy, Greece) have demonstrated lower death rates from colon and breast cancer compared to countries that consume lower amounts. Similarly, persons in the Mediterranean basin have lower risk of skin cancer development, which may result from deposition of squalene in the skin. Based on experimental and other population data, olive oil may also decrease the risk of lung and breast cancer.

Bibliography

- Owen RW, Giascosa A, Hull WE, et al. Olive-oil consumption and health: the possible role of antioxidants. Lancet Oncol 2000;1:107-111

- Owen RW, Giacosa A, Hull WE, et al. The antioxidant/anticancer potential of phenolic compounds isolated from olive oil. Eur J Cancer 2000;36:1235-1247

- Owen RW, Haubner R, Wurtele G, et al. Olives and olive oil in cancer prevention. Eur J Cancer Prev 2004;13:319-326

- Visioli F, Galli C. Biological properties of olive oil phytochemicals. Crit Rev Food Sci Nutr 2002;42:209-221

- Tripoli E, Giammanco M, Tabacchi G, et al. The phenolic compounds of olive oil: structure, biological activity, and beneficial effects on human health. Nutr Res Rev 2005;18:98-112

- Yumi ZHY, Hashim ME, Gill CIR, et al. Components of olive oil and chemoprevention of colorectal cancer. Nutr Rev 2005;63:374-386

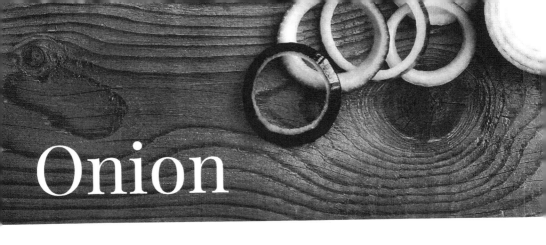

Onion

Background

Onions, *Allium cepa*, belong to the large *Allium* genus that contains garlic (*A. sativum*), leeks (*A. porrum*), and shallots (*A. ascalonicum*). These foods contain similar chemical constituents that not only impart cancer-fighting properties, but also the pungent, aromatic odor which results from organic sulfur compounds such as allylmercaptane and diallyldisulfide which, when exhaled, cause "onion breath." The "crying" or tearing that occurs while cutting raw onions results from release of propanethial S-oxide which is then converted into sulfuric acid and other irritating compounds within the tear glands.

Anticancer properties

Onions contain numerous phytonutrients that have been shown to slow or prevent cancer cell growth in laboratory rodents. Diallyl disulfide and allylcysteine inhibit growth of cancer cells and induce cancer cell death (*apoptosis*). Onions have been demonstrated in laboratory studies to inhibit cell mutations, prevent DNA damage, scavenge free radicals, and decrease cell proliferation of various cancer cells such as lung, colon, breast, prostate, and skin. The organosulfur compounds found in onions inhibit the conversion of a variety of chemicals into cancer-promoting carcinogens. Onion extracts administered to mice decreased growth of carcinogen-induced liver and colon tumors. Onion oils have slowed growth of leukemia cells.

Several epidemiologic studies strongly suggest a protective effect of onion intake against various cancers. Studies in Europe and China have shown a significantly lower risk of stomach cancer with increasing onion intake. A French and Swiss study revealed a decreased risk of breast cancer associated with regular onion ingestion. A study from China showed a 75% decreased risk of esophagus cancer with regular onion intake. Data for the prevention of colon cancer are conflicting with some studies finding a decreased risk and some showing no effect of onions. Other cancers shown to be possibly prevented by regular onion intake in epidemiology studies include lung, throat, and uterus.

Bibliography

- Bianchini F, Vainio H. *Allium* vegetables and organosulfur compounds: do they help prevent cancer? Environ Health Perspect 2001;109:893-902

- Challier B, Perarnau JM, Viel JF. Garlic, onion and cereal fibre as protective factors for breast cancer: a French case-control study. Eur J Epidemiol 1998;14:737-747

- Dorant E, van den Brandt PA, Goldbohm RA, et al. Consumption of onions and a reduced risk of stomach carcinoma. Gastroenterology 1996;110:12-20

- Hsing AW, Chokkalingam AP, Gao YT, et al. *Allium* vegetables and risk of prostate cancer: a population-based study. J Nat Cancer Inst 2002;94:1648-1651

- Setiawan VW, Yu GP, Lu QY, et al. *Allium* vegetables and stomach cancer risk in China. Asian Pac J Cancer Prev 2005;6:387-395

- Tache S, Ladam A, Corpet DE. Chemoprevention of aberrant crypt foci in the colon of rats by dietary onion. Eur J Cancer 2007;43:454-458

Oregano

Background

Oregano (*Oregano compactum* or *marjoram*) is a widely-grown aromatic plant whose leaves are an integral part of many cultures, especially the Mediterranean. Oregano is widely available in fresh and dried forms and adds a characteristic flavor to many cuisine styles. Interestingly, the Mediterranean diet, a diet rich in phytonutrients, has been associated with a lower risk of colon and other cancers. Some researchers have attributed that this may be due in-part to high consumption of oregano and other phytonutrient-rich herbs. Oregano has been used medically for its antiinflammatory effects for years, but recently researchers have studied its potential anticancer properties.

Anticancer properties

El Babili and colleagues isolated 46 compounds from oregano leaves, with carvacrol, thymol, and p-cymene accounting for approximately 90%. Other phytochemicals included the polyphenol, gallic acid, the flavonoid, quercetin, as well as anthocyanins and catechins. Extracts of oregano oil were shown to be toxic to breast cancer cells *in vitro* in several studies. Other laboratory studies have demonstrated oregano extract to inhibit growth and lead to *apoptosis* (cell death) of colon cancer cells. Inhibition of leukemia cell lines has been demonstrated when the cells were exposed to oregano extracts by down-regulation of BCL2, a protein that some cancer cells possess that leads to decreased cell death. Oregano has been shown to block numerous growth pathways in cancer cells, which may reduce the risk of cancer or hold promise for therapeutic drugs in the future.

Bibliography

- Abdel-Massih RM, Fares R, Bazzi S, et al. The *apoptotic* and antiproliferative activity of *Origanum majorana* extracts on human leukemic cell line. Leuk Res 2010;34:1052-1056

- Al-Dhahri Y, Attoub S, Arafat K, et al. Anti-metastatic and antitumor growth effects of *Origanum majorana* on highly metastatic human breast cancer cells: inhibition of NFkB signaling and reduction of nitric oxide production. PLoS One 2013;8:e68808

- Arcila-Lozano-Pina G, Lecona-Uribe S, et al. Oregano: properties, composition, and biologic activity. Arch Latinoam Nutr 2004;54:100-111

- El-babili F, Bouajila J, Souchard JP, et al. Oregano: chemical analysis and evaluation of its antimalarial, antioxidant, and cytotoxic activities. J Food Sci 2011;76:512-518

- Savini I, Arnone R, Catani MV, et al. *Origanum vulgare* induces *apoptosis* in human colon cancer caco2 cells. Nutr Cancer 2009;61:381-389

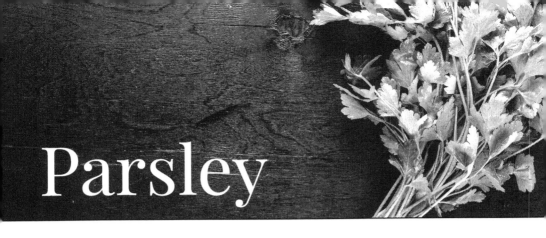

Parsley

Background

Parsley (*Petroselinum crispum*) is a green leafy plant indigenous to the Mediterreanean region that is used worldwide in many forms of cooking. In the United States, flat leaf and curly leaf parsley are widely available, although the curly variety is often presented as a garnish. Parsley is also utilized in dried form and is a convenient way of adding phytonutrients to daily cooking.

Anticancer properties

Although parsley is often used as a garnish and not consumed with a meal, this herb contains not only vitamins and minerals, but also anticancer phytochemicals such as flavonoids and antioxidants, notably apigenin. Apigenin is a flavonoid found in celery and parsley that possesses antiinflammatory, antioxidant, and anticarcinogenic properties that scavenges free radicals. Apigenin administration to mice with prostate cancer suppressed tumor growth and abolished metastasis *via* inhibition of the PIK3/AKT pathway; similar effects were noted in human prostate cancer cell lines. Similarly, one study demonstrated apigenin suppressed pancreatic cancer cell growth and induced *apoptosis in vitro* in-part by suppression of the nuclear factor *kappa beta* (NF-kB) pathway. Various laboratory studies have shown apigenin to inhibit growth of breast, cervix, colon, lung, leukemia, thyroid, and skin cancer cells. Apigenin inhibits enzymes that lead to cancer cell growth, increases intracellular glutathione (an antioxidant), and inhibits cancer cell metastasis and invasion by regulating production of various proteases. Human studies have shown that subjects fed parsley have measurable apigenin levels and evidence of increased serum levels of antioxidant enzymes.

Animal studies have shown regression of gastric cancer with apigenin administration. Epidemiological studies suggest that higher intake of apigenin and other flavonoids was inversely associated with cancer in general, and possibly cancers of the gastrointestinal and respiratory tracts.

Bibliography

- Kuo CH, Weng BC, Wu CC, et al. Apigenin has antiatrophic gastritis and antigastric cancer progression effects in *Helicobacter pylori*-infected Mongolian gerbils. J Ethnopharmacol 2014;151:1031-1039

- Meyer H, Bolarwinwa A, Wolfram G, et al. Bioavailability of apigenin from apiin-rich parsley in humans. Ann Nutr Metab 2006;50:167-172

- Patel D, Shukla S, Gupta S. Apigenin and cancer chemoprevention: progress, potential, and promise (review). Int J Oncol 2007;30:233-245

- Shukla S, Gupta S. Apigenin: a promising molecule for cancer prevention. Pharm Res 2010;27:962-978

- Wu DG, Yu P, Li JW, et al. Apigenin potentiates the growth inhibitory effects of IKK-B-mediated NF-kB activation in pancreatic cancer cells. Toxicol Lett 2014;224:157-164

Pomegranate

Background

  Pomegranate (*Punica granatum*) is an ancient fruit frequently mentioned in the Old

Testament and grows on a low-lying tree throughout Asia, the Mediterranean basin, and the

Western United States. Research on the anticancer properties of pomegranate has increased in the

last decade with this intimidating-appearing fruit possessing antioxidant, antiinflammatory, and

anticarcinogenic properties. As a result, pomegranate juice, the easiest way to ingest this fruit, is now

widely available.

Anticancer properties

  Pomegranates consist of a tough, inedible skin, an inner white and bitter pericarp, and

the aril, or seed, which contains the juice and oils. This discussion will pertain to the juice since

this is by far the most practical and easiest way to add pomegranate to the diet. Pomegranate juice

contains numerous phytochemicals with anthocyanins, (which provide the color), punicalagin,

ellagic acid, gallic acid, caffeic acid, quercetin, and epigallocatechin gallatin being among the most

widely studied and prominent constituents. Egallic acid and punicalagin, which are present in high

amounts in pomegranates, are powerful antioxidants and have been shown in laboratory studies

to decrease tumor cell growth, cause cancer cell death (*apoptosis*), and decrease the growth of new

blood vessels (angiogenesis) within tumor masses. Inhibition of the ability of cancer cells to spread,

or metastasize, has been demonstrated in laboratory experiments. Researchers have also shown that

pomegranate juice possesses more antioxidant activity than green tea. Laboratory studies have also shown juice to stop the growth of breast, prostate, colon, skin, and lung, and leukemia cancer cells in laboratory rodents. This may occur not only by an antioxidant effect, but also by blocking release of chemicals known as cytokines from normally present immune cells. Also, blockade of estrogen formation decreased the rate of breast cancer cell growth in laboratory experiments.

The best clinical data available from human studies pertain to prostate cancer, the most common cancer among men. An 8-ounce glass of commercial pomegranate juice decreased the rate of rise of prostate specific antigen (PSA) in patients with prostate cancer that recurred after surgery or radiation. Corresponding studies on these patients' blood showed evidence of decreased prostate cancer cell proliferation and increased cell death (*apoptosis*). This data suggests that pomegranate juice may become an important treatment for prostate cancer prevention or treatment in the future.

Bibliography

- Heber D. Multitargeted therapy of cancer by ellagitannins. Cancer Letters. 2008;269:262-268.

- Jurenka J. Therapeutic applications of pomegranate (*Punica granatum*): a review. Alt Med Rev 2008;13:128-144

- Khan N, Afaq F, Kweon MH, et al. Oral consumption of pomegranate fruit extract inhibits growth and progression of primary lung tumors in mice. Cancer Res 2007;67:3475-3482

- Kim ND, Mehta R, Yu W, et al. Chemopreventive and adjuvant therapeutic potential of pomegranate (*Punica granatum*) for human breast cancer. Breast Cancer Res Treat 2002;71:203-217

- Lansky EP, Newman RA. *Punica granatum* (pomegranate) and its potential for prevention and treatment of inflammation and cancer. J Ethnopharmacol 2007;109:177-206

- Pantuck AJ, Leppert JT, Zomorodian N, et al. Phase II study of pomegranate juice for men with rising prostate-specific antigen following surgery or radiation for prostate cancer. Clin Cancer Res 2006;12:4018-4026

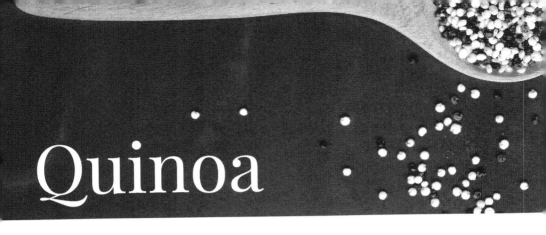

Quinoa

Background

Quinoa is an interesting food that is a species of a grain known as goosefoot (*Chenopodium quinoa*), a small shrub-like plant found worldwide. Plants of this genus are known as leaf vegetables, similar to spinach. Quinoa is actually a protein-dense grain and is gluten-free, making it a popular staple in gluten-intolerant individuals. Quinoa is native to South America in the region of the Andes mountains, first cultivated approximately 4000 years ago. Quinoa is grown widely in Chile, Bolivia, and Peru and given its nutritional properties, has been called a "superfood."

Anticancer properties

Quinoa is high in dietary fiber, which increases fecal bulk and decreases bowel transit time. It may decrease colon cancer risk by limiting contact of toxic bowel contents (e.g., bile acids) with the intestinal lining. It is high in various phytonutrients such as polyphenols and flavonoids. Rodents fed diets with quinoa seeds had decreased lipid peroxidation (which can damage cells and promote carcinogenesis) and increased antioxidant activity of blood and various tissues. Quinoa also contains significant amounts of vitamin E, which acts as an antioxidant.

Bibliography

- Abugoch JLE. Quinoa (*Chenopodium quinoa willd.*): composition, chemistry, nutritional and functional properties. Adv Food Nutr Res 2009;58:1-31

- Laus MN, Gagliardi A, Soccia M, et al. Antioxidant activity of free and bound compounds in quinoa (*Chenopodium quinoa willd.*) seeds in comparison with durum wheat and emmer. J Food Sci 2012;77:1150-1155

- Pasko P, Barton H, Zagrodzki P, et al. Effect of diet supplemented with quinoa seeds on oxidative status in plasma and selected tissues on high fructose-fed rats. Plant Foods Hum Nutr 2010;65:146-151

- Vega-Galvez A, Miranda M, Vergara J, et al. Nutrition facts and functional potential of quinoa (*Chenopodium quinoa willd.*), an ancient Andean grain: a review. J Sci Food Agric 2010;90:2541-2547

Rosemary

Background

Rosemary *(Rosmarinus officinalis)* is a woody-stemmed plant that produces fragrant leaves that are utilized worldwide to add a pungent, yet pleasant, flavor to many dishes. Rosemary can be used fresh, but is often dried, which makes it readily available. This herb has recently been noted to contain various compounds that have been shown to promote health and possibly prevent cancer.

Anticancer properties

Rosemary is commonly used in Mediterranean cooking, and has been shown to possibly decrease risk of cancer if ingested regularly. This herb contains potent antioxidants known as diterpenes, such as carnosol. Carnosol has been demonstrated to have anticancer properties such as inhibition of cell differentiation, proliferation, and migration as well as promotion of *apoptosis* (cell death). Laboratory studies have demonstrated that carnosol extracts from rosemary inhibit breast, leukemia, prostate, melanoma, and lung cancer cell lines. Other laboratory data have shown carnosol to induce cell cycle arrest and block various signaling pathways in prostate cancer cells (e.g., PIK3/AKT pathway). There also may be an additive anticancer effect of carnosol when ingested with curcumin, which is found in turmeric. The phenolic compound rosmarinic acid also possesses antioxidant activity and may contribute to the anticancer effects of rosemary. A case-control study in Italy revealed a trend for a decreased risk of lung cancer in persons who regularly consumed rosemary.

Bibliography

- Al-Sereiti MR, Abu-Amer KM, Sen P. Pharmacology of rosemary (*Rosmarinus officinalis* Linn.) and its therapeutic potentials. Indian J Exp Biol 1999;37:124-130

- Fortes C, Forastiere F, Farchi S, et al. The protective effect of the Mediterranean diet on lung cancer. Nutr Cancer 2003;46:30-37

- Johnson JJ. Carnosol: a promising anticancer and anti-inflammatory agent. Cancer Lett 2011;305:1-7

- Lopez-Jimenez A, Garcia-Caballero M, Medina MA, et al. Anti-angiogenic properties of carnosol and carnosic acid, two major dietary compounds from rosemary. Eur J Nutr 2013;52:85-95

- Ngo SNT, Williams DB, Head RJ. Rosemary and cancer prevention: preclinical perspectives. Crit Rev Food Sci Nutr 2011;51:946-954

- Yesil-Celiktas O, Sevimli C, Bedir E, et al. Inhibitory effects of rosemary extracts, carnosic and rosmarinic acid on the growth of various human cancer cell lines. Plant Foods Hum Nutr 2010;65:158-163

Sunflower Seeds

Background

Sunflower seed is the fruit of the sunflower, *Helianthus annuus*. Sunflower oil is found within the seeds, or the edible portion known as the kernel or heart. Commonly available sunflower seeds are either black or striped black and white. They are cultivated and eaten in a variety of ways worldwide, especially the Mediterranean, Middle East, and North America. Sunflower seeds may be eaten roasted, raw, or added to salads and various main dishes. The oil is obtained by pressing the seeds and is widely available for culinary use.

Anticancer properties

Sunflower seeds and oil contain the essential fatty acid, linoleic acid, fiber, and the antioxidant, vitamin E. Sunflower seed oil has been demonstrated to block experimentally-induced abdominal tumors in mice. Researchers believe that linoleic acid inhibits carcinogenesis and tumor formation and has been shown to block breast cancer cell growth in rodents. Linoleic acid has also been demonstrated to modulate the immune response to cancer cells and stimulate activated macrophages to kill tumor cells. Sunflower seed extracts possess antioxidant capacity as demonstrated on various assays that assess free radical scavenging properties. Decreased growth of HeLa and glioma (brain tumor) cells were noted in one study. A population-based study in Germany showed that postmenopausal women who consumed sunflower seeds had a lower risk of developing breast cancer compared to those with no intake.

Bibliography

- Hubbard NE, Lim D, Erickson LK. Effect of separate conjugated linoleic acid isomers on murine mammary tumorigenesis. Cancer Lett 2003;190:13-19

- Silva LA, Nascimento KAF, Maciel MCG, et al. Sunflower seed oil-enriched product can inhibit Ehrlich solid tumor growth in mice. Chemotherapy 2006;52:91-94

- Zaineddin AK, Buck K, Vrieling A, et al. The association between dietary lignans, phytoestrogen-rich foods, and fiber intake and postmenopausal breast cancer risk: a German case-control study. Nutr Cancer 2012;64:652-665

- Zhang XC, Shao HL, Wang JX, et al. Purification and characterization of an inhibitor of a cathepsin B-like proteinase from sunflower seed. J Enzyme Inhib Med Chem 2006;21:433-439

- Ziboh VA, Miller CC, Cho Y. Metabolism of polyunsaturated fatty acids by skin epidermal enzymes: generation of anti-inflammatory and anti-proliferative metabolites. Am J Clin Nutr 2000;71:361S-366S

Tomato Paste

Background

Tomato, *Lycopersicon* species, is actually a fruit and is one of the most versatile as well as healthful foods available. Tomatoes are widely available year-round in fresh, canned, sun-dried, and frozen forms. Lycopene, an abundant caretenoid pigment responsible for the red color of tomatoes, is the most well-studied anticancer phytochemical in tomatoes and will be the focus of this discussion.

Anticancer properties

Tomatoes contain lycopene, a carotenoid pigment similar to vitamin A, that imparts the red and orange colors. Lycopene is the most abundant carotenoid in human plasma and, being lipophilic (fat-soluble), concentrates within the adrenal glands, liver, and prostate. Lycopene is a potent antioxidant that has been experimentally demonstrated to protect cells from damage by free-radicals. Lycopene may also decrease cancer cell growth, induce cell death (*apoptosis*), and protect cells from DNA damage. Importantly, heating of tomatoes increases the ability of lycopene to be utilized by the body. Products such as ketchup, tomato paste, and tomato sauce are an especially rich and concentrated source of lycopene. Ripening increases lycopene content. A variety of laboratory studies have demonstrated that lycopene slows or prevents growth of breast, lung, leukemia, liver, and prostate cancer cells. Lycopene also may increase the ability of immune cells known as T-helper cells to attack cancer cells.

Observational studies have demonstrated a lower risk of prostate cancer in men with higher blood-levels of lycopene. For instance, the Physicians' Health Study, a very large long-term study of healthy U.S. male physicians, demonstrated that men who eventually developed prostate cancer had lower average blood lycopene levels than those men who did not. Other studies have shown similar results: a lower blood level of lycopene is associated with a higher risk of prostate cancer. An intake of ten or more weekly servings of tomato products may reduce the risk of prostate cancer by approximately 35%. A study of elderly people from Massachusetts demonstrated that a high long-term intake of tomato products was associated with a 50% decrease in death from cancer in general. Other studies have shown that tomato intake and high lycopene levels may decrease the risk of cancers of the breast, prostate, stomach, and lung.

Bibliography

- Agarwal S, Rao AV. Tomato lycopene and its role in human health and chronic diseases. Can Med Assoc J 2000;163:739-744

- Gann PH, Ma J, Giovannucci E, Willett W, et al. Lower prostate cancer risk in men with elevated plasma lycopene levels: results of a prospective analysis. Cancer Res 1999;59:1225-1230

- Giovannucci E, Ascherio A, Rimm EB, et al. Intake of carotenoids and retinol in relation to risk of prostate cancer. J Nat Cancer Inst 1995;87:1767-1776

- Miller EC, Giovannuci E, Erdman W, et al. Tomato products, lycopene, and prostate cancer risk. Urol Clin North Am 2002;29:83-93

- Rao AV, Agarwal S. Role of antioxidant lycopene in cancer and heart disease. J Am Coll Nutr 2000;19:563-569

- Rao AV, Fleshner N, Agarwal S. Serum and tissue lycopene and biomarkers of oxidation in prostate cancer patients. Nutr Cancer 1999;33:159-164

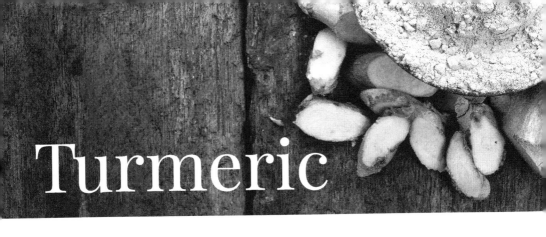

Turmeric

Background

Turmeric (*Curcuma longa*) is a rhizome belonging to the ginger family and when dried and ground, forms a deep orange-yellow powder that is used in a variety of cuisines. Turmeric has been utilized for hundreds of years in India and surrounding countries not only as a food spice and fabric dye, but also for medicinal purposes. It is one of the most researched spices due to the nutraceutical potential of its most active biologic constituent, curcumin. In fact, much research has been carried out at the M.D. Anderson Cancer Center in Houston on curcumin and its potential to not only prevent, but also treat, a variety of cancers.

Anticancer properties

There is significant published data that show curcumin suppresses oxidative cell damage, inflammation, and amyloid (an abnormal protein that interferes with cell function) formation. Additionally, curcumin possesses numerous biologic properties that make it a potential inhibitor of cancer growth and even a potential therapeutic agent. A discussion of the numerous biologic intracellular targets of curcumin is well beyond the scope of this discussion, but it has been shown to inhibit transcription factors (e.g., NF-kB), growth factors (e.g., EGFR, VEGFR), protein kinases (e.g., PIK3) and mediators of inflammation (e.g., TNF, COX). In fact, curcumin inhibits many of the molecular pathways that current anticancer drugs used in humans target (e.g., EGFR by cetuximab, RAS by vemurafenib, BCR-ABL by imatinib, and mTOR by everolimus). Modulation or inhibition of these targets is responsible for curcumin's pro-*apoptotic* (cell-death causing), antiinflammatory, antiangiogenic, and antiproliferative effects on neoplastic cells. Curcumin also has been shown to decrease the invasive and metastatic potential of cancer cells in laboratory experiments.

Interestingly, consumption of spices (including turmeric) is felt to contribute to the much lower incidence of colorectal cancer in India as compared to the United States. Many clinical trials have involved curcumin administration to patients with a variety of cancers, producing varied results with no dose-limiting toxicity. An important observation in many trials is that curcumin is not readily absorbed from the gastrointestinal tract and that black pepper enhances absorption significantly. As such, turmeric and black pepper should be ingested together, which in addition to increasing curcumin absorption, may also act synergistically in regards to antioxidant benefit. A variety of studies suggest that curcumin can suppress growth of cancer cells from a variety of organs including the brain, breast, esophagus, stomach, colon, head and neck region, liver, lung, prostate, pancreas, ovary, and skin. It seems that addition of significant amounts of turmeric to the diet may help decrease the risk of various cancers without undue toxicity; however, it should administered with black pepper to enhance absorption.

Bibliography

- Aggarwal BB, Harikumar KB. Potential therapeutic effects of curcumin, the anti-inflammatory agent, against neurodegenerative, cardiovascular, pulmonary, metabolic, autoimmune, and neoplastic disease. Int J Biochem Cell Biol 2009;41:40-59

- Anand P, Sundaram C Jhurani S, et al. Curcumin and cancer: an "old-age" disease with an "age-old" solution. Cancer Lett 2008;261:133-164

- Sung B, Prasad S, Yadav VR, et al. Cancer cell signaling pathways targeted by spice-derived nutraceuticals. Nutr Cancer 2012;64:173-197

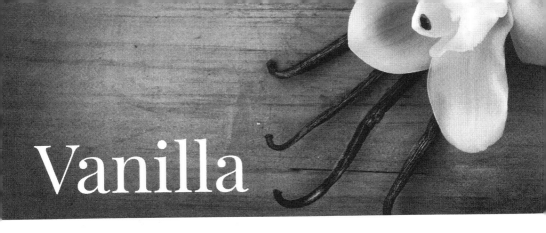

Vanilla

Background

Vanilla is a flavorful extract from orchids of the genus *Vanilla*, most often from the Mexican species, *V. planifolia*. The word vanilla literally means "little pod" and it is in these pods that the very small vanilla beans reside. Vanilla was historically only grown in Mexico and Central America because it required an indigenous bee for pollination; technology has overcome this and now vanilla is grown globally. Vanilla is the second most expensive spice following saffron, since it takes much labor to grow and harvest the pods. Nonetheless, vanilla imparts a wonderful flavor to a variety of cuisines, notably desserts. Recently, attention has been paid to a potential anticancer agent found in vanilla known as vanillin.

Anticancer properties

Vanilla contains a variety of phytonutrients, the most abundant being vanillin, which is responsible for the scent and flavor. Vanillin has been found to possess anticancer properties such as repair of DNA mutations. Vanillin induced cell death (*apoptosis*) of human colon cancer and cervical cancer (HeLa) cell lines and also caused arrest of cell growth. Other researchers have shown that vanillin inhibits a key pathway in cancer cell growth known as NF-kB *in vitro* and reduced the number of lung metastases in mice with breast cancer. Tumor blood vessel growth (angiogenesis) was suppressed as well as a key cancer cell growth pathway known as the PIK3 pathway in laboratory studies.

Bibliography

- Hazen J. Vanilla. Chronicle Books, 1995.

- Liang JA, Wu SL, Lo HY, et al. Vanillin inhibits matrix metalloproteinase-9 expression through down-regulation of nuclear factor-kappa B signaling pathway in human hepatocellular carcinoma cells. Mol Pharmacol 2009;75:151-157

- Lirdprapomongkol K, Kramb JP, Suthiphongchai T, et al. Vanillin suppresses metastatic potential of human cancer cells through PI3K inhibition and decreases angiogenesis in vivo. J Agric Food Chem 2009;57:3055-3063

- Lirdprapomongkol K, Sakurai H, Kawasaki N, et al. Vanillin suppresses *in vitro* invasion and *in vivo* metastasis of mouse breast cancer cells. Eur J Pharm Sci 2005;25:57-65

- Lirdprapomongkol K, Sakurai H, Suzuki S, et al. Vanillin enhances TRAIL-induced apoptosis in cancer cells through inhibition of NF-kappa B activation. *In Vivo* 2010;24:501-506

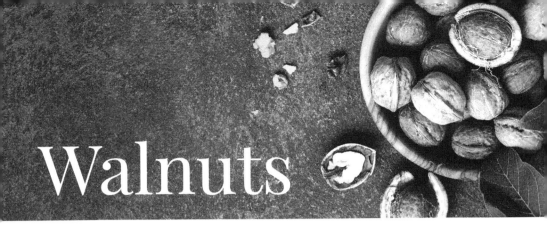

Walnuts

Background

The walnut is the seed of trees of the genus *Juglans* of which common species include the English walnut (which originated in Persia) and the eastern black walnut (which is native to the Eastern United States). Walnuts are round, single-seed fruits of the walnut tree, known as stone fruits. Walnuts are grown worldwide, with China being the top producer.

Anticancer properties

Walnuts are very dense in a variety of nutrients including amino acids, fat, and fiber. Additionally, walnuts possess the polyunsaturated fatty acids linolenic acid and linoleic acid. These fatty acids promote health by their antioxidant and antiinflammatory effects and may prevent cardiovascular disease and cancer. Phytosterols from walnuts have been shown to decrease proliferation of breast cancer cells *in vitro*. The chemical, juglone, inhibited the growth and increased *apoptosis* (cell death) of HeLa cancer cells in one study. Extracts from walnuts also have been shown to inhibit growth of human colon, prostate, and kidney cancer cell lines.

154

Bibliography

- Carvalho M, Ferreira PJ, Mendes VS, et al. Human cancer cell antiproliferative and antioxidant activities of *Juglans regia* L. Food Chem Toxicol 2010;48:441-447

- Reiter RJ, Tan DX, Manchester LC, et al. A walnut-enriched diet reduces the growth of LNCaP human prostate cancer xenografts in nude mice. Cancer Invest 2013;31:365-373

- Vanden Heuvel JP, Belda BJ, Hannon DB, et al. Mechanistic examination of walnuts in prevention of breast cancer. Nutr Cancer 2012;64:1078-1086

- Zhang W, Liu A, Li Y, et al. Anticancer activity and mechanism of juglone on human cervical carcinoma HeLa cells. Can J Physiol Pharmacol 2012;90:1553-1558

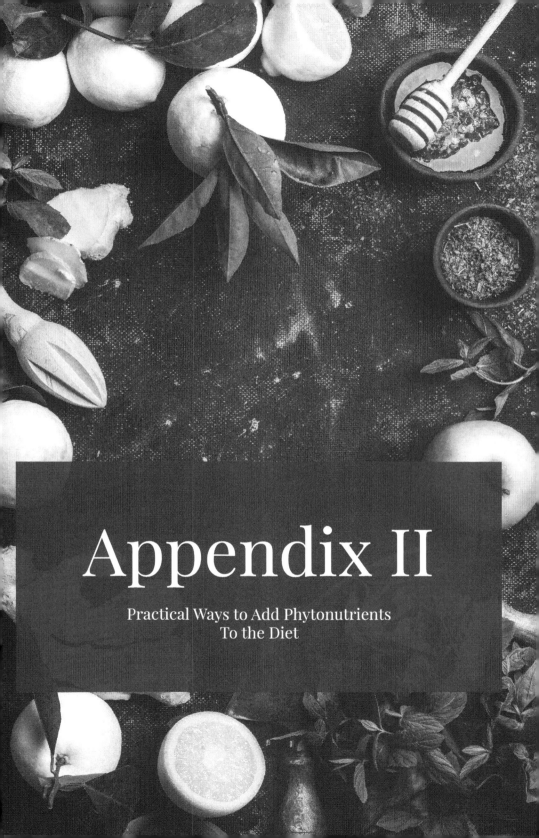

Appendix II

Practical Ways to Add Phytonutrients
To the Diet

Throughout this book, the concept of adopting a lifestyle of healthy plant-based eating is presented as a superior way of maintaining health as opposed to "dieting," adopting food fads, or taking supplements. In my opinion, and, based on the literature ,there is no "one size fits all" when it comes to diet. That being stated, however, the Mediterranean style of diet does have ample data published in the medical literature to adopt as a basic framework for one's individual dietary pattern. Additionally, incorporating elements of dietary practices from India and Japan is also important. For example, many Indian spices are rich in phytonutrients that have been shown experimentally to suppress cancer cell formation, growth, and spread. Curcumin found in turmeric is perhaps the most widely studied and potent anticancer agent; however, other Indian spices that may decrease cancer risk include fennel seed, cumin, coriander, and peppercorn to name a few (the reader is referred to *Appendix 1* for specific details on these spices). Japanese people frequently enjoy longevity, and some have attributed this to a high intake of mustard seed which is widely used in their cuisine.

As such, "*metronomic phytonutrition*" is not necessarily a strict diet based on any one culture. Rather, this concept of eating as an attempt to decrease cancer risk, is based on adopting a diet that *consistently* includes a variety of phytonutrient-rich foods — no matter the culture of origin. Since there are numerous vegetables, fruits, seeds, herbs, and spices that literally contain thousands of phytonutrients, an individual can create their own personal eating style based on taste and availability of ingredients. If one likes Mediterranean food, then a diet that regularly includes tomato products, olive oil, garlic, oregano, basil, and parsley would be a good start. If one enjoys Mexican or Southwest-style food, addition of cumin and chili peppers is a good option. People who enjoy the pungency and aromatic nature of Indian food may add turmeric, fennel seed, and cumin to their diet in liberal fashion. People with no particular dietary style can basically limit red meat and ingest a variety of fruits and vegetables seasoned with a number of the herbs and spices discussed in *Appendix 1*. Extra virgin olive oil adds many benefits as well. In my personal cooking, I lean heavily Mediterranean, using large amounts of garlic, EVOO, and tomato products; however, I often add in Indian spices such as turmeric , black pepper, and cumin to increase the phytonutrient content. To be sure, there is no *one* way to cook and enjoy the taste of food.

Below are a few simple and practical ways to increase daily phytonutrient intake.

Breakfast

- Fruit-based smoothies containing blueberries, apple, citrus peel, green tea, kale, and flaxseed (the possibilities are unlimited and based on personal taste and access to a quality blender; please see *Appendix 1* for phytonutrient-rich foods to add to your smoothie)

- Add turmeric, black pepper, cumin, chili powder, and fresh or dried herbs to eggs—with a dash of EVOO

- Add ground flaxseed, orange peel, and cinnamon to pancakes and waffles; drizzle with pure maple syrup instead of refined sugar-saturated, commercial, high glycemic-index syrup

Lunch

- Add kale to salad and drizzle with EVOO; top with herbs and phytonutrient-rich sunflower or flax seeds and spices as noted in *Appendix 1* to suit your taste

- Add colorful vegetables to salad (or eat individually)

- Consume fruits, such as apples or blueberries

- Drink iced green tea without sweetener; could add coconut sugar since does contain antioxidants and has a lower glycemic index than table sugar

Dinner

- Add phytonutrient-rich spices and herbs (consider making a blend of your dried favorites and keep in a jar) to EVOO and use to dip whole-grain bread into instead of butter or margarine

- Consume salad daily enriched with kale and colorful vegetables and sprinkled with phytonutrient-rich herbs and spices; make a vinaigrette dressing from EVOO and lemon or orange juice with citrus peel

- Roast vegetables such as carrots in EVOO; top with black pepper and/or spices and herbs of choice

- Drink iced green tea with lemon

Snacks

- Limit refined flour and sugar; baked goods made with whole grains, flaxseed, nuts, seeds, dark chocolate chips, and dried fruits are an excellent source of phytonutrients and have a lower glycemic index than prepared sweet snacks, such as cookies or pastry

- Dried berries, raisins, and nuts/seeds are portable and quick

- Fresh fruits, especially apples, are easy to transport and loaded with phytonutrients (remember, "an apple a day keeps the doctor away")

- Fresh vegetables, especially carrots and celery (an underappreciated food that contains the valuable phytonutrient, apigenin)

Beverages

- Filtered water with lemon/citrus peel

- Green tea (excellent source of antioxidants, especially catechins)

- Coffee (contains numerous phytochemicals)

- Skim milk with dark cocoa powder (rich in polyphenols)

- Tomato juice (rich in lycopene)

- Pomegranate juice (rich in punicalagin)

About the Author

Mark Marinella, MD, FACP is a full-time, practicing medical oncologist in Dayton, Ohio and is board-certified in Medical Oncology and Internal Medicine by the American Board of Internal Medicine. He is as a member of the American Society of Clinical Oncology and received his Doctor of Medicine Degree from Wright State University School of Medicine. He completed an Internal Medicine Residency at the University of Michigan Medical Center and a Fellowship in Medical Oncology at Wright State University School of Medicine. He is an Assistant Clinical Professor of Internal Medicine at Wright State University School of Medicine, where he is involved with the Hematology-Oncology Fellowship. He is chair of the Oncology Committee at Miami Valley Hospital. Dr. Marinella treats all types of adult cancers with a special interest in lymphoma, blood cancers, breast cancer, gastrointestinal cancer, and prostate cancer. He is the author of dozens of various articles in the medical literature and six books including *Tarascon Oncologica* and *Handbook of Cancer Emergencies*, both published by Jones and Bartlett.

Dr. Marinella has a special interest in nutrition in hospitalized and critically ill patients and previously was a Certified Nutrition Support Physician (CNSP). He has a clinical interest in the role that nutrition plays in patients with active cancer as well as those who are cancer survivors. Due to his interest in cancer medicine, nutrition, and cooking Mediterranean food, he began researching the published medical studies on cancer in Mediterranean countries. It was this combination of interests that led to writing this book.

86939686R00099

Made in the USA
Lexington, KY
18 April 2018